D1451022

Lasers in Cardiovascular Disease

Rodney A. White, M.D.
Associate Professor of Surgery
UCLA School of Medicine
Los Angeles, California
Chief, Vascular Surgery
Harbor-UCLA Medical Center
Torrance, California

Warren S. Grundfest, M.D.
Assistant Professor of Surgery
UCLA School of Medicine
Assistant Director of Surgery
Cedars-Sinai Medical Center
Los Angeles, California

YEAR BOOK MEDICAL PUBLISHERS, INC.

Chicago • London • Boca Raton

1 2 3 4 5 6 7 8 9 0 KC 91 90 89 88 87

Library of Congress Cataloging-in-Publication Data

White, Rodney A.
    Lasers in cardiovascular disease.
    Includes bibliographies and index.
    1. Cardiovascular system—Surgery. 2. Lasers in surgery. I. Grundfest, Warren
S. II. Title. [DNLM: 1. Cardiovascular Diseases—therapy. 2. Lasers—therapeutic use.
WG 166 W5873L]
RD597.W47   1987   617'.41'059   87-15977
ISBN 0-8151-9258-4

Sponsoring Editor: Daniel J. Doody
Associate Managing Editor: Deborah Thorp
Production Project Manager: Carol A. Reynolds
Proofroom Supervisor: Shirley E. Taylor

*THIS BOOK IS DEDICATED TO THOSE
WHO STRIVE TO IMPROVE THE QUALITY
OF LIFE*

Contributors

Robert F. Bonner, Ph.D.
Senior Physicist, Biomedical Engineering and Instrumentation Branch, Division of Research Services, National Institutes of Health, Bethesda, Maryland

Alan W. Cole
Director of Communications, Harbor-UCLA Medical Center, Torrance, California

D. Lynn Doyle, M.D., F.R.C.S.(C.)
Clinical Assistant Professor, Department of Surgery, University of British Columbia; Health Sciences Center Hospital, Vancouver, British Columbia

John Eugene, M.D.
Assistant Professor of Surgery, University of California at Irvine, Irvine, California

James S. Forrester, M.D.
Professor of Medicine, UCLA School of Medicine; Director, Cardiovascular Research, Cedars-Sinai Medical Center, Los Angeles, California

Warren S. Grundfest, M.D.
Assistant Professor of Surgery, UCLA School of Medicine; Assistant Director of Surgery, Cedars-Sinai Medical Center, Los Angeles, California

Stanley R. Klein, M.D.
Assistant Professor of Surgery and Anatomy, UCLA School of Medicine, Los Angeles, California; Department of Surgery, Harbor-UCLA Medical Center, Torrance, California

George Kopchok, B.S.
Biomedical Engineer, Director, Experimental Laser Laboratory, Harbor-UCLA Medical Center, Torrance, California

James B. Laudenslager, Ph.D.
Supervisor, Laser Physics and Applications Group, Jet Propulsion Laboratory, California Institute of Technology, Pasadena, California

Martin B. Leon, M.D.
Senior Investigator and Co-Director, Cardiac Catheterization Laboratory, Cardiology Branch, National Heart, Lung, and Blood Institute, National Institutes of Health, Bethesda, Maryland

Frank I. Litvack, M.D.
Assistant Professor of Medicine, UCLA School of Medicine; Associate Director, Cardiac Catheterization Laboratory, Cedars-Sinai Medical Center, Los Angeles, California

Thomas L. Robertson, M.D.
Chief, Cardiac Diseases Branch, Division of Heart and Vascular Diseases, National Heart, Lung, and Blood Institute, National Institutes of Health, Bethesda, Maryland

Timothy A. Sanborn, M.D.
Associate Professor of Medicine, Boston University School of Medicine; Associate Visiting Physician, University Hospital, Boston, Massachusetts

Paul D. Smith, Ph.D.
National Institutes of Health, Bethesda, Maryland

Jouni Uitto, M.D., Ph.D.
Professor and Chairman, Department of Dermatology, Thomas Jefferson University, Philadelphia, Pennsylvania

Geoffrey H. White, M.D., F.R.A.C.S.

Assistant Professor of Surgery, UCLA School of Medicine; Chief, Vascular Surgery, Veterans Administration Wadsworth Medical Center, Los Angeles, California; Vascular Surgeon, Harbor-UCLA Medical Center, Torrance, California

Rodney A. White, M.D.

Associate Professor of Surgery, UCLA School of Medicine, Los Angeles, California; Chief, Vascular Surgery, Harbor-UCLA Medical Center, Torrance, California

Preface

The use of lasers in medicine and surgery has generated significant interest. The initial enthusiasm was based mainly on the fascination for a "star-wars" concept, which ascribes mystical powers to this unique form of energy. The idea that a laser can be used as a surgical instrument to cut tissue, destroy tumors, and open obliterated atherosclerotic arteries triggered a degree of speculation and enthusiasm that preceded the reality that scientists and physicians have been trying to determine. This effort has required the development of a unique collaboration among physicists, engineers, biologists, and clinicians. To the pleasant surprise of all, many of the speculations regarding the potential uses of lasers in medicine are rapidly developing into applications.

The adaptation of lasers as therapy for cardiovascular diseases is in its infancy, but the use of lasers to treat difficult clinical problems and improve overall care of patients is coming close to reality. The ability to selectively ablate abnormal tissues and atherosclerotic lesions and enhance the technical accuracy and healing of vascular repairs is now more than an appealing concept.

The objective of this book is to convey a basic understanding of laser physics, safety, and laser-tissue interactions, and to describe the current state-of-the-art and eminent developments to physicians, allied health professionals, and those interested in the frontiers of medicine. It will become evident that the current laser applications are not the cure-all that the extensive publicity may lead one to believe; in a curious way the field is developing in a manner that adds credence to some of the early speculations regarding the use of laser surgery.

RODNEY A. WHITE, M.D.
WARREN S. GRUNDFEST, M.D.

Acknowledgments

We wish to thank the contributors for their timely assistance in the preparation of this book. Special thanks are given to Deanna Alford for her editing and secretarial skills, and to Alan Cole for the majority of the graphics and artwork in the text, including the logo(s). Both individuals made an invaluable contribution. Special thanks are also given to our colleagues, research associates, and support personnel at Harbor-UCLA and Cedars-Sinai Medical Centers, who consistently provided help and encouragement during the preparation of this book. Carol Reynolds, Daniel Doody, and Fran Perveiler of Year Book Medical Publishers, Inc., were also extremely helpful and supportive.

RODNEY A. WHITE, M.D.
WARREN S. GRUNDFEST, M.D.

Contents

Color Plates

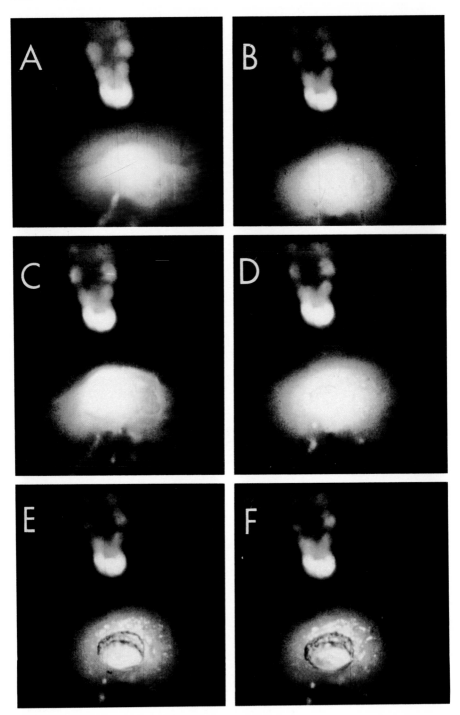

Plate 1.—See legend at top of facing page.

←

Plate 1.—A, this frame is obtained from the high-speed filming of Nd:YAG ablation of athero-sclerotic tissue at 30 W delivered via a 400-μm fiber. The white light is the aiming light of the laser. The laser irradiation begins, and approximately 0.25 seconds later the tissue begins to turn white. **B,** at 0.4 seconds a small crater begins to form. As the crater enlarges, one can see material melt and boil. **C,** boiling can sometimes occur explosively as deeper and deeper layers of tissue are heated. Note that laterally the tissue is thermally injured and it blanches and turns white. **D,** as all molten material evaporates, temperature rises and pyrolysis begins. The crater is easily visible, with sharply defined margins. However, denaturation of the protein laterally turns the tissue from pink to gray. **E,** as pyrolysis continues, carbonization begins and the crater walls turn black. **F,** as temperatures rise laterally, molten material pours back into the crater, now filling the base of it. As the crater cools, lateral thermal effects extend outward.

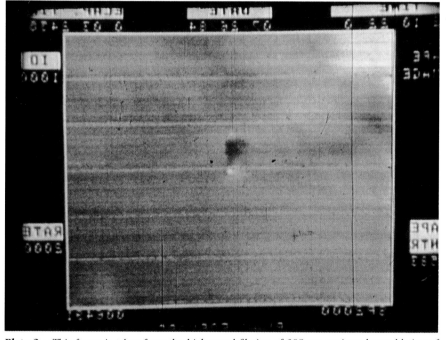

Plate 2.—This frame is taken from the high-speed filming of 308-nm excimer laser ablation of atherosclerotic tissue. The beam is directed from the laser output mirror and is 0.4 × 0.8 mm. Pulse duration is 80 nanoseconds. The area of tissue ablation is also 0.4 × 0.8 mm. The ambient light is coming in at a 45-degree angle. No debris is observed escaping from the crater, and the incision has extremely sharp, precisely cut edges. There are no surrounding tissue effects. The color or the texture of the tissue do not change.

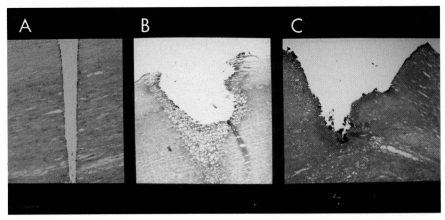

Plate 3.—A comparison of the histologic effects of three different lasers on atherosclerotic aorta. **A** shows a cut made with an excimer laser from a fiberoptic waveguide. This cut is in human atherosclerotic aorta. The thickness of the aorta here is approximately 2.2 mm. The width at the very top is 0.4 mm, and the average width is approximately 0.35 mm. The crater walls are sharp, without carbonization or blast damage. A 2-μm rim of eosinophilic tissue is present, but adjacent tissue is not affected. **B** shows the effects of an Nd:YAG laser, again ablating atherosclerotic tissue that is only minimally calcified. The fiberoptic waveguide is aimed perpendicular to the intimal aortic surface. Spot size was 0.9 mm in diameter. The crater is 2.1 mm in diameter by approximately 1.8 mm in depth; note the surrounding zone of vacuolized tissue, carbonized edges, and loss of tissue architecture. **C** shows a histologic section of human cadaver atherosclerotic aorta after irradiation with an argon laser using a 0.4-mm fiberoptic waveguide with the energy set at 8 W, spot size 0.5 mm. The crater created was 2.2 mm in diameter by approximately 1.6 mm in depth. Note the carbonization and lateral coagulation injury. (From Grundfest WS, Litvak F, Glick D, et al: Current status and future prospects for angioscopy and laser angioplasty. *J Vasc Surg* 1987; 5:667–672. Reproduced by permission.)

Plate 4.—This is a four-panel histologic comparison of the ablation effects at four wavelengths. **A** shows the effect of Nd:YAG ablation at 1,060 nm at 7 nanoseconds (nsec), 100 mJ/sq mm. There is significant charring and surrounding blast damage to the tissue. **B** shows the effect of 532 nm, or green light, similar to that from the argon laser, but pulsed at 7 nsec at 65 mJ/sq mm. This wavelength produced variable effects and significant blast damage and, in some cases, shredded the tissue. At higher energy densities both of these lasers were able to cut tissue. However, the energy was so high that it cut the quartz plates used to hold the tissue as well. **C** shows the effect of 353 nm at 7 nsec, 45 mJ/sq mm. Note that there are visible thermal effects at this wavelength. However, they are small compared with the continuous-wave lasers; the edges are not as smooth as those obtained in the shorter wavelength. **D**, in contrast, shows 266 nm at 7 nsec, 11 mJ/sq mm, which produced extremely precise edges with minimal thermal damage. The shorter the ultraviolet wavelength, the more precise the ablative process for this particular tissue. (From Grundfest WS, Litvak F, Goldenberg T, et al: Pulsed ultraviolet lasers and the potential for safe laser angioplasty. *Am J Surg* 1985; 150:220–226. Reproduced by permission.)

$\longrightarrow$

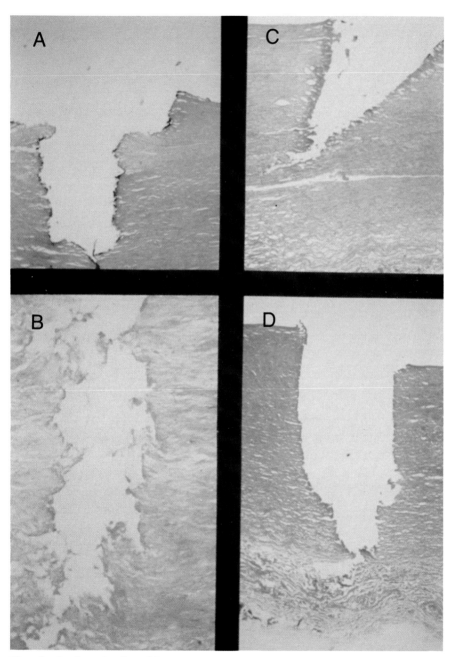

Plate 4.—See legend at foot of facing page.

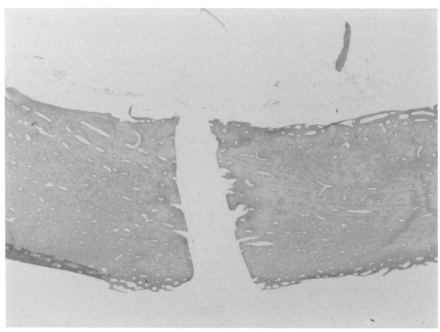

Plate 5.—This 4-mm-thick section of bovine femur was irradiated at 308 nm output from a 1.0-mm fiberoptic waveguide, carving a 1-mm channel. This channel was created in approximately 1 minute 45 seconds with a laser operating at 20 Hz. Fiberoptic output was 75 mJ/sq mm. (From Litvak F, Grundfest WS, Beeder C, et al: Laser angioplasty: Status and prospects. *Semin Intervent Radiol* 1986; 3:75–81. Reproduced by permission.)

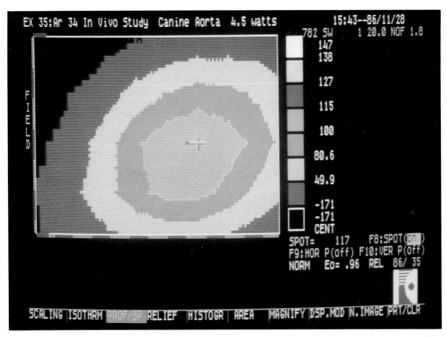

Plate 6.—Computer-generated color thermogram of argon ablation of normal canine aorta (intimal surface). The red area is the hottest, the blue, the coolest. The crosshairs in the frame denote the maximum temperature of 117° C.

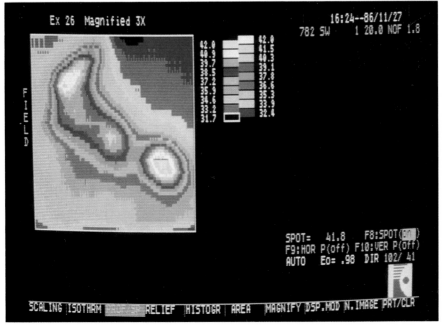

Plate 7.—Computer-generated thermogram shows excimer irradiation at 31.5 mJ/sq mm per pulse. The maximal temperature in this frame was 41.8° C; three consecutive pulses are visible, with the last pulse having the highest temperature.

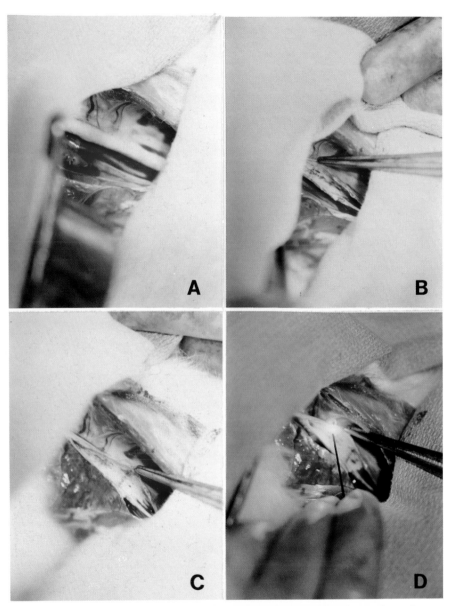

Plate 8.—Argon ion laser endarterectomy in an atherosclerotic rabbit. **A,** an atherosclerotic rabbit aorta. The aorta is markedly thickened and discolored chalk white. **B,** a longitudinal arteriotomy is made to expose an atheroma. **C,** lines of laser craters have been created at one end of the atheroma. **D,** individual argon ion laser exposures are being used to create lines of laser craters at the other end of the atheroma. (From Eugene JA, McColgan SJ, Hammer-Wilson M, et al: Laser endarterectomy. *Lasers Surg Med* 1985; 5:265–274. Reproduced by permission.)

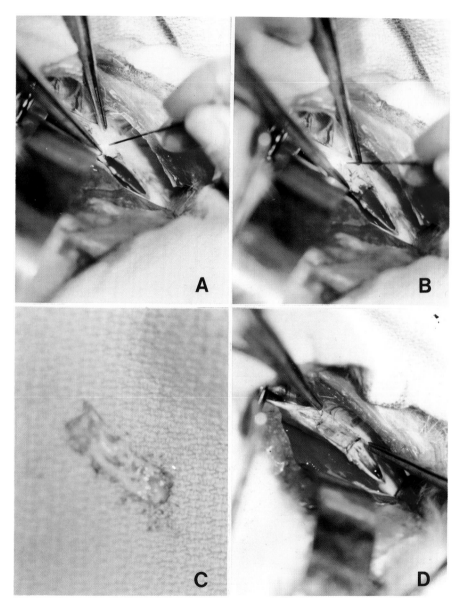

Plate 9.—Argon laser endarterectomy in an atherosclerotic rabbit. **A,** the atheroma is being elevated away from the aorta by continuous argon ion laser radiation. **B,** the cleavage plane is being developed within the media by continuous argon ion laser radiation. **C,** the atheroma has been removed from the artery. **D,** the completed endarterectomy has a smooth, glistening surface with proximal and distal end points welded in place. (From Eugene JA, McColgan SJ, Hammer-Wilson M, et al: Laser endarterectomy. *Lasers Surg Med* 1985; 5:265–274. Reproduced by permission.)

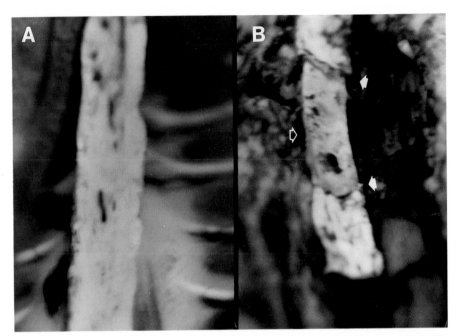

Plate 10.—The luminal surface of an atherosclerotic aorta 48 hours after injection of Photofrin II, 5 mg/kg. **A,** the porphyrin-laden atherosclerotic plaque fluoresces salmon-pink when photographed under ultraviolet light. **B,** following open laser endarterectomy with an argon ion laser, the endarterectomy surface *(open arrow)* lacks gross fluorescence, whereas the residual plaque beyond the end points *(closed arrow)* retains fluorescence.

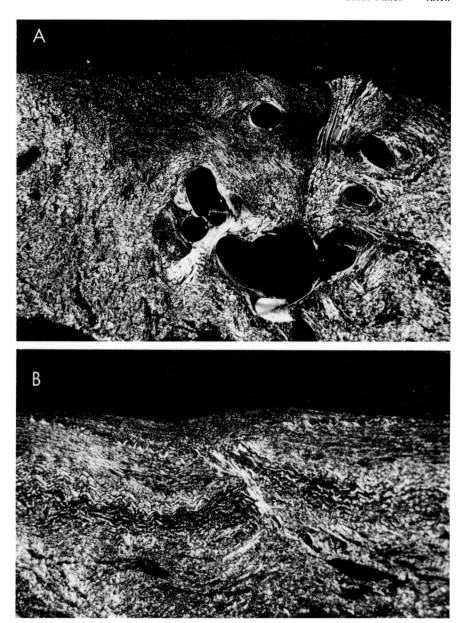

Plate 11.—Histologic appearance of sutured (**A**) and argon laser–welded (**B**) arteriotomies at 4 weeks. The disorientation of the collagen, elastin, and cellular matrix in the sutured repair in contrast to the near-normal restoration of the arterial wall architecture in the laser-welded specimen is highlighted by a Sirius red stain viewed under polarized light (× 40). (Histologic sections and photographs compliments of James Anderson, M.D., Ph.D., Case Western Reserve University, Cleveland.)

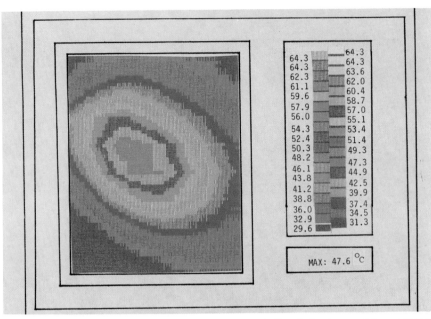

Plate 12.—Computerized thermographs at the anastomotic line during laser welding at 0.50 W, demonstrating the effect of saline irrigation. In this instance, the tissue heated to 47.6° C with application of laser light.

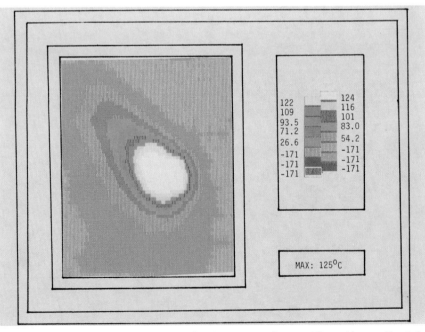

Plate 13.—Temperatures in excess of 125° C during argon laser welding without saline irrigation at 0.50 W power.

1

Introduction

George Kopchok, B.S.
Rodney A. White, M.D.

The recent development of lasers for use in medicine and surgery has created a new frontier with numerous potential cardiovascular applications. Among the questions to consider while exploring this new technology are (1) Why use lasers to treat cardiovascular diseases? (2) What are the special considerations required for choosing appropriate instrumentation, assuring facility safety, and conducting personnel training?

Lasers are expensive equipment that have unique space and facility requirements. Unless they fulfill a need in our armamentarium that is not available by current, less expensive technologies, the use of lasers in cardiovascular medicine is not appropriate. As outlined in the remainder of this text, there are several advantages that lasers offer to the cardiovascular surgeon, cardiologist, and radiologist. Specific ablation of intracardiac and intravascular lesions, disobliteration of totally occluded small-internal-diameter arteries, augmentation of current clinical techniques such as percutaneous balloon dilatation, and laser welding of vascular tissue are current applications that may soon find significant clinical utility. The initial studies using balloon angioplasty were performed less than a decade ago, but this technique is now used widely for rapidly expanding indications. Laser surgery appears to have the same potential for broad applicability and development.

CHOICE OF MEDICAL LASER SYSTEMS

In most cases the lasers that are currently available in hospitals are improperly designed or have inadequate power ranges to make them easily adaptable to cardiovascular applications. Because of the expense of purchasing and maintaining lasers, hospitals are obviously concerned with maximizing the

1

use and cost-effectiveness of new instruments. A new laser system that is to be used primarily for cardiovascular applications should have the broadest applicability to multiple specialties. The desirability of any particular instrument directly increases with its versatility.

Conceptually, the ideal laser should be an instrument that can be dialed over a wide power range (watts), is tunable over the entire spectrum of wavelengths, that permits fiberoptic transmission, and is designed to accommodate any future demands placed on the instrument. Unfortunately, at the present state of technology, lasers that meet these specifications are not available.

Currently, carbon dioxide (CO_2) (10,600nm), neodymium:yttrium-aluminum-garnet (Nd:YAG) (1,060 nm), and argon (488 to 515 nm) are the clinical lasers available at most hospitals. Carbon dioxide lasers have power outputs of a few hundred milliwatts to 100 W and are used for cutting or ablating soft tissue. The Nd:YAG lasers are most reliable between 1 and 60 W and are used by general surgeons and gastroenterologists for tissue coagulation. Argon lasers provide a steady output from the milliwatt to 15-W level and are used primarily in ophthalmology and dermatology to coagulate pigmented lesions. The energy from argon and Nd:YAG lasers are transmitted through flexible quartz optic fibers, whereas CO_2, because of its wavelength, is transmitted through a microscope, through an articulating arm, or potentially by a hollow waveguide. Although other promising laser prototypes are at various stages of experimental development, none at present is commercially available for cardiovascular applications. Throughout this interval of rapid development, one must keep in mind the current availability of lasers and separate that from what may be state-of-the-art in the future.

ORGANIZATION AND PERSONNEL

To make rational decisions regarding lasers, laser safety protocols and laser acquisition should be scrutinized and controlled by a hospital laser committee. Key individuals who should be involved in the committee activities are administrative personnel, the hospital safety officer, a representative from the hospital mechanical services, a representative from nursing, and a representative from each of the medical and surgical subspecialties that have an interest in laser applications. Frequent meetings of this group are necessary to assess the current state of laser applications within the hospital, to evaluate the priorities in laser program development, and to assess the utility and cost-effectiveness of proposed new purchases.

An administrative representative to the laser committee is obviously essential to evaluate the cost-effective use of instrumentation and to represent the priorities in hospital program development. It is also administrative responsibility to address billing for laser procedures. Most of the cardiovascular laser applications are still considered experimental, and third-party payers may refuse payment on this basis. Some of these procedures are done as adjuncts to other standard procedures, such as laser-assisted balloon angioplasty, which could further complicate the reimbursement process. In other instances, the laser procedures may significantly reduce the cost of therapies that currently have a substantial diagnosis-related group fee.

The laser safety officer fulfills an important role on the laser committee by establishing a laser safety protocol for the institution and by ensuring that instrumentation, new programs, and new facilities fulfill these requirements and are accompanied by the necessary approvals. A representative from mechanical services is needed to evaluate the power and plumbing requirements for new instrumentation and to expedite facility construction. Nursing plays a key role in space planning, training, equipment maintenance, and oversight of the safe use of the lasers.

The final responsibility for laser safety, and determining appropriate requirements for credentials to use the lasers, rests with the institutional laser safety committee. Physicians can demonstrate proficiency either by previous experience or by certification from an approved training program. Each department chairman should generate a list of approved laser treatments and decide in conjunction with the laser safety committee which procedures a particular physician can perform. Table 1–1 displays a sample format for credentialing standards.

LASER SAFETY

Establishing a laser safety protocol, facility specifications, approvals, in-services, and continuing education for personnel is essential to maintain a safely functioning facility. All laser users must receive training in facility operating procedures and precautions to prevent personal injury and property damage. Only certified personnel should be permitted to set up, use, and discontinue use of laser equipment. Although laser radiation can cause eye damage, skin burns, and combustion of flammable materials, these hazards can easily be averted by a carefully planned program.

The physician and all key laser operating room personnel should be fully versed in laser physics, nomenclature regarding laser energy, and laser tissue interactions.[1, 2] The physician user is ultimately responsible for selecting the wattage and appropriate lens or fiber for each procedure. In addition, a laser safety officer or his designee should be present during all procedures.

Laser procedure and operating rooms must have all windows covered with nontransparent barriers to prevent inadvertent passage of laser light. Access to the room should be restricted while the laser is activated. Clearly visible warning signs with flashing red lights to signify that the system is activated are mandatory. The laser should remain in the off position or with the safety shutter closed until ready for use. Control of laser emission by a pedal and direction of the beam by a hand control greatly enhance the safety. Laser energy should be directed and activated only when it is aimed at a specific target.

TABLE 1–1.
Credentialing Standards

A. Laser safety standards and practices should be developed and explored by a hospital laser safety committee (subcommittee of the hospital's safety committee). The primary responsibility for laser safety should be organized by an individual designated by the institution and approved by the committee as the laser safety officer.
B. Department chairmen or their selected representatives within the department or division hold the responsibility to ensure that the use of lasers on their service is performed by competent personnel. Staff members shall petition for permission to use lasers through their department chairman or department/divisional representatives.
C. Staff members desiring to utilize the laser must be trained in the use, care, and physics of the laser and have fulfilled the following criteria:
   1. The candidate has demonstrated proficiency, knowledge, and safety in the use of lasers through previous use, which is common knowledge of the department chairman or his representative and the laser safety committee.
   2. The candidate may present certification of approved training sessions indicating that the staff member has completed a laser course of at least 4 hrs of didactic and 2 hrs of clinical "hands-on" experience. The applicant should also demonstrate proficiency specific to that physician's specialty by observation of a departmental preceptor for two or more procedures, if necessary, based on the preceptor's decision. Documentation of the preceptor's approval should be on file.
D. The department chairman will forward all approved laser use requests to the chairman of the laser safety committee for proficiency verification and activation to user status.
E. "Active laser use status" staff members will receive a copy of the hospital's laser safety guidelines and will acknowledge their reading and understanding of these guidelines by signing a copy of the laser standards of practice, which will be kept on file in the department chairman's office and/or in the facility where the laser is being used (e.g., operating room).
F. Each department chairman, by generating a list of laser treatments within his specialty, shall document which procedures the petitioning physician shall have permission to perform. When appropriate, privileges that are limited to the use of particular type(s) of laser(s) should be noted. The laser safety committee has the final responsibility for ensuring appropriate and safe use of laser devices.

Control of fiberoptic laser delivery is similar to the use of electrocautery in that the system is activated only when it is in contact with the tissue being treated. Reflective surgical instruments should be avoided and reflective surfaces in the laser procedure room minimized. Moist sponges in the operating field can prevent combustion of dry or paper materials.

Due to focusing effects of the cornea and lens of the eye, radiant exposure can be amplified 100,000 times at the retina.[3] Careless misdirection of the laser light even at low powers can result in instantaneous burning of the retina and consequent blindness. Everyone in the operating room, including the patient, must have appropriate eyewear during the procedures. For the CO_2 laser, clear plastic lenses are adequate, and wet gauze can be used to protect the patient's eyes. Green lenses (nontransparent to 1,060 nm) are recommended for the Nd:YAG laser, and amber lenses (nontransparent to 488 to 515 nm) are necessary to absorb the green or blue light of the argon laser. Other lasers with different wavelengths require specific lenses for eye protection as recommended by the manufacturer.

Lasers are classified according to their potential to cause biologic injury. The parameters used for laser classification are laser power, wavelength, exposure duration, and beam spot size at the area of interest. Lasers are stratified into four classes. Class I, or exempt lasers, produce no hazard under normal

---

Laser Standards of Practice

This form is used to provide written verification that the user has been advised of all safety precautions and operational hazards. Laser operators are responsible for assuring that the operational requirements described in this document are followed during procedures.

I. Operational guidelines
   A. Prior to beginning any laser procedure, the laser safety officer and the user must be sure that:
      1. There are no flammable chemicals in the room.
      2. Opaque barriers are intact to prevent propagation outside the controlled access area.
      3. There is adequate ventilation to eliminate hazardous concentration of by-products if plastics or combustibles are used in the procedure.
      4. Warning signs on the entrance door and laser, and English labels on laser controls, are intact.
      5. The entrance door to the controlled area is secured.
   B. During procedures:
      1. Appropriate protective eyewear must be worn by all personnel and by the patient.
      2. User must be sure that laser beam path is free of specularly reflective surfaces and combustible materials and that the beam is terminated in a noncombustible, nonreflective barrier.
      3. Lasers are to be activated, when possible, by pedal control and directed to the operative site by hand pieces to maximize accuracy and safety.
   C. Following laser operative procedures:
      1. Laser is to be turned off before controlled access entrance is opened.
      2. Key to the laser control is to be removed when the laser is not in use to prevent unauthorized operation.
      3. Laser operating entrance is to be locked at all times when the facility is not in use, or the instrumentation must be secured in some way to prevent unauthorized use.

_____

User Signature

FIG 1–1.
Pertinent guidelines and procedures for standards of practice in laser use.

operating conditions. The total amount of energy produced is less than the maximum permissible exposure level, and therefore no special facility or safety precautions are needed. Class II lasers are low-power lasers that do not present a visual hazard. The eye normally closes in approximately 0.25 seconds when exposed to a noxious stimulus. This response avoids eye damage from a class II laser. Class IIIa lasers operate with maximum power output of 5 mW or less and power density of 2.5 mW/sq cm or less. These lasers present a hazard if viewed through any collecting optics but present no hazard if viewed momentarily with the unaided eye. Class IIIb lasers can damage the eyes if viewed directly but present no hazard to the skin. Class IV denotes high-power laser systems that are hazardous to the eyes, skin, and flammable material from a direct and/or diffusely reflected beam. Facility requirements vary with the class of laser being used. Generally, class IV lasers are used in cardiovascular surgical applications, and therefore facilities must be in accordance with requirements for this classification.[2, 4]

The most frequent cause of laser injury in industrial environments is electrical accidents. Activation of the laser systems frequently requires high current; thus, the electrical outlets should be carefully positioned when the room is designed. Adequate warning signs and in-service training are essential to prevent inadvertent accidents. The laser system should be stored so that components and ignition keys are secured when the laser is not being used. Figure 1–1 summarizes the pertinent guidelines and procedures that should be included in a laser standards of practice.

REFERENCES

1. Arndt KA, Noe JM, Northam BC, et al: Laser therapy—Basic concepts and nomenclature. *J Am Acad Dermatol* 1981; 5:649–654.
2. *American National Standard for the Safe Use of Lasers.* New York, American National Standards Institute, 1980, ANSI Z-136.1.
3. *Laser Safety Guide.* Toledo, Ohio, Laser Institute of America, 1986.
4. *A Guide for the Control of Laser Hazards.* Cincinnati, American Conference of Governmental Industrial Hygienists, 1981.

2

Laser Fundamentals

James B. Laudenslager, Ph.D.

The word *laser* is an acronym for *l*ight *a*mplification by *s*timulated *e*mission of *r*adiation. To most people a laser is a device that generates a highly directional beam of monochromatic light (i.e., a single color), and this beam of laser light can produce intense power densities on a target at considerable distances from the laser source. These characteristics of a laser beam are quite different from those of light generated from conventional sources, such as incandescent lights, fluorescent lights, or the light produced by chemical combustion reactions in a candle flame or an oil lamp. Conventional light sources, although ideal for illumination, produce light with a wide distribution of frequencies or colors, and the light scatters in all directions; consequently, the light energy reaching a target at a distance drops off inversely as the square of the distance between the target and the light source.

Lasers currently used in medical applications cover wavelength regions in the ultraviolet, visible, and infrared portions of the electromagnetic spectrum (Fig 2–1), which is nonionizing to tissue. The history of laser devices is recent, although the fundamental principles of lasers are based on the development of quantum theory in the early 1900s. The first laser demonstrated was the visible ruby laser by Maiman in 1959,[1] followed by the helium-neon (He-Ne) laser by Javan et al. in 1961,[2] the visible argon ion laser,[3] metal ion laser,[4] and infrared carbon dioxide (CO_2) laser in 1964,[5] and the ultraviolet discharge excimer (meaning excited dimer) laser in 1975,[6–8] to list only a few. Historically, a laser device usually has a 9- to 10-year development period from the time it is first demonstrated until the time it is adequately engineered and packaged into a reliable system for various applications. This long gestation period is one reason for the recent increased utilization of lasers in medical applications, particularly for argon ion, neodymium:yttrium-aluminum-garnet (Nd:YAG) and CO_2 lasers, which have had the most extensive engineering period.

Common features of lasers currently used by medical practitioners[9] are (1) they are expensive; (2) the devices are complex and require specialized maintenance; (3) the laser technology is in a constant state of evolution and

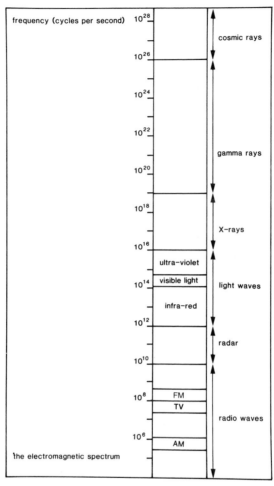

FIG 2–1.
The electromagnetic spectrum. The frequency region for laser radiation is from 10^{12} to 10^{16} cps.

improvement; and (4) medical lasers (>1 W) require specialized power outlets and water cooling, consume an appreciable amount of valuable operating room space for all the associated equipment, and require protective eye measures to shield personnel from the laser radiation. Despite these factors, the use of controlled laser light has found important applications in many disciplines of medical treatment. The following chapters will present several emerging applications for laser treatment of cardiovascular disease.

Often, a physician will ask why scientists and engineers cannot eliminate these negatives from laser devices, particularly the high costs. Why is a laser that is powerful enough to cut through bone not reduced to the size of a wristwatch or hand calculator, as is often depicted in movies? The technical reasons for the size and for the requirements of water cooling and specialized power will be better understood once the principles of the laser device are explained. The high cost of medical lasers is due in part to the relatively short time span the laser has been available for use in medical treatment coupled with the lengthy period required for engineering these devices for reliable usage. Also, the lack of understanding of the interaction of laser radiation with tissue has led to improper choice of laser parameters for a variety of medical applications. Because of these factors, there is not yet a large demand for lasers; hence, they are manufactured in limited numbers, a major hindrance to lower prices.

One barrier to the wider use of lasers in medicine, as well as other areas of laser application, is the tendency to associate the laser device with the application in a generic manner without understanding the nature of the laser energy interaction on the material or tissue being irradiated. Even researchers who deal with laser development often use the term *laser* generically instead of identifying the parameters of the beam of light used for the particular application in terms of (1) power density, (2) wavelength, (3) spatial and temporal properties, and (4) total accumulated energy dosage.

To illustrate, precise ablation of atherosclerotic plaque has been demonstrated using an ultraviolet xenon chloride (XeCl) excimer laser with fiber delivery without thermal damage to surrounding tissue.[10] The common assumption is that the use of an XeCl excimer laser with fiberoptic delivery is the key to achieving the desired clinical result. However, this is not the case! The key factors in achieving precise cutting without thermal damage are the application of pulsed ultraviolet laser with optimal parameters. Careful studies in our laboratory have shown that this can be achieved with pulsed ultraviolet lasers delivered through a fiberoptic with (1) a pulse duration on the order of 100 nanoseconds (a nanosecond [nsec] is one billionth of a second) but less than 1 μsec; (2) an energy density or fluence at the distal end of the fiber of greater than 20 mJ/sq mm per pulse but less than 100 mJ/sq mm; (3) a wavelength near 300 nm; and (4) a pulse repetition frequency of 20 pulses per second (pps). If the same XeCl excimer laser were used under different operating conditions with a pulse energy of less than 5 mJ/sq mm of energy exiting from the distal end of the fiber, the tissue would show signs of thermal damage with irregular rather than precisely cut edges, even though it was the same laser at the same wavelength. Additionally, if the pulse energy from the XeCl laser were the same as in the favorable case but the pulse width were only 10 ns, the fiberoptic would be easily damaged, even though the same energy density was used. If a continuous wave (CW) laser operating in this ultraviolet wavelength region were used at a power level that would cut the tissue and would be transmitted through the fiber, one would produce severe thermal damage to the tissue even though the wavelength was still in the ultraviolet. If a high pulse repetition rate of 500 pps or very high focused energy density of 1 J/sq mm were used to irradiate the tissue, it would produce severe blast damage. For each laser procedure and tissue, an optimal set of parameters must be defined!

For these reasons there is no universal laser device or set of laser light parameters for effective treatment of all medical diseases, just as there is no universal drug for all human disorders.

Therefore, greater acceptance of lasers for medical treatment will come with better understanding of the proper choice of laser light energy values needed to perform a specific treatment. When this knowledge is identified from careful scientific studies in the research laboratory, a safely packaged laser device and delivery system operated within the appropriate range of conditions will greatly increase the acceptance of lasers to clinical applications.

LASER FUNDAMENTALS

A laser device inefficiently converts electrical energy into light energy. Energy in the form of a laser beam of light energy has certain special characteristics compared with other forms of energy. Before understanding the laser device, one requires an understanding of some properties and characteristics of light. Light is electromagnetic radiation that has a frequency, phase, and amplitude. Light also has particle characteristics, and a beam of light consists of discrete packets of energy called photons. To understand medical laser applications it is important to understand that light is a form of radiant energy that is convertible into other forms of energy, such as electrical, heat, chemical, and kinetic energy. From quantum theory, the energy of a photon of light is related to its frequency of oscillation in the electromagnetic spectrum, which

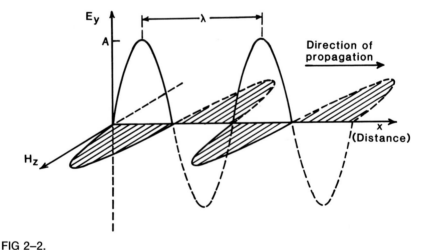

FIG 2–2.
The instantaneous electric (E_y) and magnetic (H_z) field strength vectors of a light wave with wavelength (λ) as a function of position along the axis of propagation (x). A is the amplitude of the electric field.

TABLE 2–1.
Various Medical Lasers and Their Properties

LASER	WAVELENGTH, μM	FREQUENCY, CPS	ENERGY/PHOTON		PHOTONS/W (J/SEC)
			J	eV	
CO_2	10.6	2.8×10^{13}	1.9×10^{-20}	0.12	3.7×10^{19}
Nd:YAG	1.06	2.8×10^{14}	1.9×10^{-19}	1.2	5.3×10^{18}
Second harmonic	0.532	5.6×10^{14}	3.6×10^{-19}	2.3	2.7×10^{18}
Third harmonic	0.353	8.4×10^{14}	5.6×10^{-19}	3.5	1.8×10^{18}
Fourth harmonic	0.266	1.1×10^{15}	7.5×20^{-19}	4.7	1.3×10^{18}
Argon ion	0.514	1.1×10^{14}	3.8×10^{-19}	2.4	2.6×10^{18}
Excimer					
XeCl	0.308	9.7×10^{14}	6.5×10^{-19}	4.0	1.6×10^{18}
XeF	0.351	8.6×10^{14}	5.6×10^{-19}	3.5	1.8×10^{18}
KrF	0.248	1.2×10^{15}	8×10^{-19}	5.0	1.3×10^{18}
ArF	0.193	1.6×10^{15}	1.0×10^{-18}	6.4	9.7×10^{17}

is in the range of 10^{12} to 10^{16} cps. These frequencies are so high that they are extremely difficult to measure experimentally, and therefore another wave property, the wavelength, or the distance between wave crests of the wave, is measured, as depicted in Figure 2–2. The wavelength is related to the speed of light *(c)* and the frequency of the electromagnetic radiation by the relationship $\lambda = c/v$, where λ is the wavelength expressed in units of length, typically angstroms (10^{-8} cm), nanometers (10^{-9} m), or microns (10^{-6} m). The energy carried by a photon of light is given by the relationship $E = hv$ or $E = hc/\lambda$, where E is a unit of energy, typically in joules, and h (Planck's constant) is 6.6 $\times 10^{-34}$ joule-seconds. To achieve a better understanding of the relationship between laser wavelength, energy of a photon, frequency, and the form of energy emanating from lasers used in medical research, Table 2–1 lists several commonly used lasers with these relationships. From the relationships in this table one can see that when the frequency of light increases, the energy per photon increases and the wavelength decreases.

Interaction of Laser Radiation With Matter

Light interacts with matter by the processes of absorption, transmission, reflection, refraction, diffraction, and several types of scattering. From common experience, we visualize objects that do not emit light of their own but reflect light from some other source of illumination, such as the sun or a lamp. Visible light covers the wavelength region from 400 to 700 nm, and white light is made up of a distribution of wavelengths in this range. When an object appears colored under illumination by white light, it is due to selective absorption of light of the colors other than that observed. The absorption of light of the other frequencies is most often converted into heat in the absorbing material.

Atoms and molecules are the chemical building blocks of matter and can exist in many different energy states. An atom has translational energy or energy of motion that is characteristic of the temperature of the environment wherein the atom is located. Atoms also have various electronic energy states in which they can exist where the electrons orbiting around the positive nucleus can be excited to higher energy orbits by absorption of a photon of radiation or by collision with a fast-moving particle such as an electron. Molecules have similar energy states of translational motion as well as numerous electronic energy states but they also absorb energy into rotational and vibrational motion, as depicted in Figure 2–3. From quantum theory, the energy levels of rotation and vibration of molecules and the electronic energy levels of atoms and molecules can have only certain discrete energy values, whereas translational motion energy can have a continuum of values. Each discrete energy level is unique to the particular atom or molecule and is the basis of the characteristic chemical properties of atoms and molecules. For an atom or molecule to absorb a photon of light to transfer it from one optically allowed energy level to another, excited energy level, the frequency of the photon must be in resonance or correspond to the exact energy difference between two energy levels in the molecular or atomic species. The majority of atoms and molecules have optical energy resonances only in the infrared and ultraviolet region of the electromagnetic spectrum. Resonances in the visible region lie between 1.5 and 3 eV, which is too high an energy for molecular rotation and

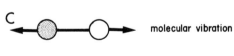

A ⬤⟶   translation

B   molecular rotation

FIG 2–3.
Pictorial view of the types of energy on atomic and molecular levels. **A** through **C** are examples of thermal motion of the molecule. **D** shows how electronic excitation can, in a molecular system, lead to direct fragmentation of chemical bonds.

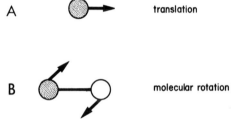

C   molecular vibration

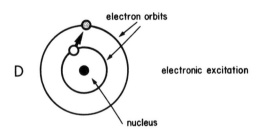

electron orbits

D   electronic excitation

nucleus

TABLE 2–2.
Characteristics of Molecules at Different Energy Levels

ENERGY TRANSITION	TYPICAL ENERGY SEPARATION, eV	SPECTRAL REGION	
		μm	FREQUENCY RANGE
Electronic	≥2.5	≤0.496	Visible → ultraviolet
Vibrational	0.12	10.3	Infrared
Rotational	1.2×10^{-3}	1,033	Radar
Translational (1 kT at 300° K)	2.6×10^{-2}	47.7	Infrared

vibration and too low an energy for most electronic excitation. However, there are certain complicated organic and inorganic molecules that do have visible resonances, and these compounds are usually designated dye molecules or pigments. Table 2–2 lists various energy transitions of atomic and molecular species with the typical magnitude of the difference between two types of energy levels and their corresponding energy spectral resonances.

Therefore, absorption of light by an irradiated material results directly in increasing the energy content of the material. This increased energy can be eliminated by reradiation of the absorbed photon; if the photon emitted has the same energy as the photon absorbed, there is no net increase in the energy of the material. If the absorbed photon is not reemitted or a photon with less energy than that absorbed is reemitted, as is usually the case, some energy remains, which is usually converted into thermal motion or heat in the absorber. For most surgical applications of laser light, the absorption process is most critical to the desired treatment.

Refraction and Reflection of Light

If a beam of light is not absorbed in a material or reflected from its surface, it is transmitted through the medium, but its path may be deviated and dispersed. When light encounters an interface between two transparent media in which the velocity is different (i.e., materials having different values of the index of refraction, such as an air-glass interface), a portion of the beam of light is reflected, and that portion that is transmitted can undergo a change in direction or is said to be refracted. We make use of this property when we focus a laser beam by means of a lens or when we disperse wavelengths using a prism. The amount of light reflected vs. transmitted is wavelength dependent and is also dependent on the angle of incidence to the medium. For example, a beam of visible light impinging perpendicular to a glass window will have a 4% reflection loss at each air-glass interface or suffer an 8% loss of beam intensity on passing through a transparent window or lens. If the same beam of light is incident at a glancing angle, the reflection loss may be less than 4% per surface, with the minimum reflection loss being defined as Brewster's angle, which is about 54 degrees for visible wavelengths incident on an air-glass interface.

Light incident on a surface can also be reflected. When the reflected portion is a substantial portion of the incident light, the surface is called a mirror. Specular reflection occurs at a smooth surface, and the reflected light returns at an angle equal to the angle of incidence of the light beam on the mirror surface. Diffuse reflection occurs at irregular surfaces, and the reflected light is dispersed in an angular distribution proportional to the cosine of the angle of incidence. This type of scattering is called lamberton scattering, after Lambert's cosine law.

Absorption and Scattering of Light

When light is absorbed, the medium that does the absorption is increased in energy content by the energy contained by the total number of photons that were absorbed. This usually results in raising the temperature of the absorbing medium. The relationship between the absorption and transmission of monochromatic light by any homogeneous, isotroptic medium obeys the Beer-Lambert formula: $I = I_o \exp(-\mu x)$, where I is the intensity of light transmitted through a dilute homogeneous medium of length x, with an attenuation coefficient of μ, and I_o is the incident intensity of the light beam. The ratio of I/I_o is the transmittance through a medium; a ratio of 1 would indicate a totally transparent medium with no absorption (this neglects reflection losses at the container surface). The formula states that for the conditions specified above for an absorbing medium, the attenuation of light is exponential, with the proportion of light absorbed per unit of length being constant.

Scattering of a beam of light by a medium does not always result in increasing the energy content of the medium and raising its temperature. Scattering of light by particles smaller than the wavelength of the light beam is called Rayleigh scattering, and its effect on a parallel beam of light is to disperse a portion of the beam in other directions. This type of scattering is strongest for shorter wavelengths, such as the ultraviolet. This scattering is symmetric in both forward and backward directions to the line of propagation of the light beam. If the scattering particles are larger in size than the characteristic of the wavelength of light (e.g., for green light, 0.4-μm diameter), the scattering is called Mie scattering and depends on the size and the shape of the particles as well as the wavelength of light. Forward scattering predominates for Mie scattering. For a laser beam propagating across a room, Rayleigh scattering is produced by the molecules of air, whereas Mie scattering results from dust or particulates in the room. When the particles are much larger than the wavelength of light, Mie scattering and diffraction dominate over Rayleigh scattering. For this reason, when smoke is placed in a laser beam path, it allows the observer to photograph its propagation across a room.

Since a laser produces energy in the form of a beam of light, the propagation of this form of energy through various media is very important in determining the effect of the light energy when it is finally incident on a tissue surface. To get a beam of light from a laser to the tissue site for a medical procedure, the process of reflection is used to steer the beam from the source to the target. Refraction or reflection from a curved surface is used to focus or defocus the spot size of the laser beam to either increase or decrease the energy and power density on the target. Fiberoptic transmission is another form of light beam propagation through an optical fiber guide by means of total internal reflection. Once the beam is delivered and shaped by the various optical elements, the processes of absorption and scattering in the target and any fluid media surrounding the target are of utmost importance in understanding the therapeutic effect of light energy.

In actuality, the simple formulas of Beer's law and Mie and Rayleigh scattering do not hold rigorously for high-energy light densities as are often used in laser procedures on tissue. First, tissue is heterogeneous, and scattering phenomena can be multiple rather than single, as occurs for low-density absorbing and scattering medium. Additionally, the high peak power generated by pulsed laser radiation often produces nonlinear absorption processes that do not occur when low-power light sources are used. For cardiovascular applications inside a blood vessel, not only may a beam of laser light be very strongly absorbed by blood itself, but the red blood cells will scatter the light or tend to defocus it by Mie scattering and diffraction. On the other hand, infrared laser beams will be strongly attenuated by water absorption and will not propagate through any aqueous media.

Stimulated Emission

Figure 2–4 shows the typical processes of light reflection, absorption, and transmission through a medium. Stimulated emission, the basis for laser action, is a special case where incident light on a specially prepared active medium results in an amplified or more intense beam of collimated light as it propagates through this amplifying medium. What Figure 2–4 does not show is the other energy source that must be used to take a normal transmitting or absorbing medium into an amplifying state. The deposition of raw electrical energy into a medium to produce an optical amplifier is the basis for a laser generator.

To illustrate the physics underlying a laser gain medium, we will consider a gaseous laser medium, although liquid, solid, and plasma media are also suitable for laser action. Table 2–2 listed the various energy values pertinent to a gaseous molecule. When a gaseous system is contained at a particular temperature and does not have any input from any other energy source, the molecules will reside in the lowest energy levels consistent with the temperature of the gas. At this equilibrium temperature, the ratio of the number of molecules in an excited state 1 to that in a lower energy state 0, with an energy difference between the two states of ΔE ($E_1 - E_0$), is given by the formula

$$n_1/n_0 = g_1/g_0 \exp - (\Delta E/KT),$$

where g_1 and g_0 are the degeneracies of each energy state. Considering the energy levels in Table 2–2, at room temperature, the fraction of molecules

LIGHT ABSORPTION AND STIMULATED EMISSION

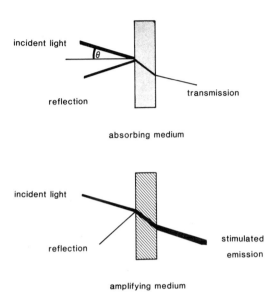

FIG 2–4.
The upper figure displays the typical effects of a beam of light incident on a typical absorbing medium. The lower figure shows the process when the medium is activated to produce stimulated emission.

existing in an excited electronic energy level is 10^{-41}, for vibrational energy the ratio is 10^{-2}, and for rotational it is 0.95. At room temperature, the probability of finding any molecules in an excited electronic state are extremely small; about 1% of the molecules reside in the first excited vibrational state, and there is almost an equal population between the lowest and next higher rotational energy states.

Possible interactions of a photon with an atom or molecule are depicted in Figure 2–5. When a photon whose energy is in resonance between two energy levels of molecular species passes through the gas, it will most probably be absorbed, since at equilibrium almost all the molecules are in the lower energy state. Therefore, the interaction of the photon with molecules at the lower energy state is to excite molecules in this lower energy state to the higher state. This process results in energy deposition into the gas. This excited species can lose this absorbed energy by reemitting a photon in a random direction. This process is called spontaneous emission. However, if by some means one can excite the gas so that there is a greater population in the excited energy level than in the lower energy level, then when the photon passes through this excited gas medium it will stimulate the emission of a photon in phase and in the same direction as the incident photon to cause the excited molecule to return to the lower energy level. This process, stimulated emission, will continue as long as a critical population difference remains between the number of molecules in the excited state and the number in the lower state. However, as stimulated emission or laser action begins, it removes molecules from the upper level and increases the population of the lower level. At some point the population difference between the two levels will decrease and the probability of a photon being absorbed will increase and cease laser action. To prevent the laser action of the gain medium from being terminated, either some means must be found to pump the lower level to the upper level at a rate faster than the depopulation by stimulated emission to the lower level, or some means is needed to depopulate the lower level at a rate faster than it is being produced by the lasing action.

Thus, the process of producing laser action is to excite a gain medium to produce either a continuous population inversion between an excited energy

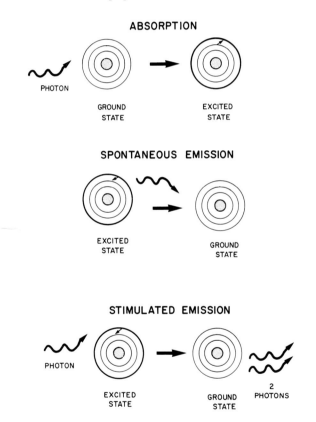

FIG 2–5.
The upper figure shows a typical atomic absorption process for a photon resulting in excitation of an electron to a higher energy level. The atom will lose the energy in collision with another species, increasing the thermal energy, or reemit the energy by spontaneous emission. Stimulated emission occurs when a photon encounters an excited state and induces the excited level to a lower level, with the emission of a photon with the same energy, phase, and direction as the incident photon.

level and a lower energy state or a temporary inversion between two levels for pulsed operation. As shown in Figure 2–6 for a three- and four-level pumping scheme, it is much easier to produce and maintain a population inversion in a multilevel system than in a two-level system, with the lower level being the ground level because the ground level is highly populated.

Figure 2–7 illustrates the processes occurring in a laser when this population inversion is produced. A gain medium is terminated with a totally reflective mirror and a partially reflective mirror. Next, energy is deposited into the gain medium to produce a high population of energetically excited species. The excited species try to lose this extra energy either by degradation of the absorbed energy into thermal motion or heat or by reradiation of the excess energy from the excited state to the lower state by spontaneous emission, which occurs with a random phase and in a random direction. Some of this spontaneously emitted light will propagate in line with the optical cavity axis and be returned through the gain medium. If the photons emitted are incident on a gas molecule in the lower energy level, they will be absorbed and more excited molecules will be produced. However, if they encounter molecules in the excited state, they will stimulate them to emit photons in the same direction, with the same energy and the same phase as the incident photons. If the pumping means maintains this excited condition, the stimulated emission process will build an intense beam of collimated light that will compete with the spontaneous emission process and the thermal degradation mechanism for deexcitation of the excited state. Essentially, the laser action is initiated from the spontaneous emission process and, rapidly using optical feedback, builds to be the dominant process for removal of excited species from the gain medium. To produce infrared laser action, a population inversion must be established between two vibrational-rotational levels, whereas to produce a visible or ultraviolet laser action, a population inversion must be produced between two electronic energy levels.

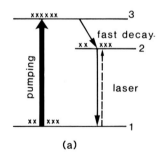

(a)

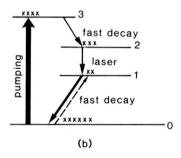

(b)

FIG 2–6.
A, schematic diagram of a three-energy-level laser pumping scheme, where a population inversion between levels 2 and 1 is required for lasing; if the pumping rate from 1 to 3 is not greater than the deactivation rate of 2 to 1, absorption as depicted in the dashed line will terminate the laser action. **B,** a four-energy-level pumping scheme, where a population inversion between levels 2 and 1 must be maintained.

EVENTS IN A LASER RESONATOR

PARTIAL
MIRROR   MIRROR

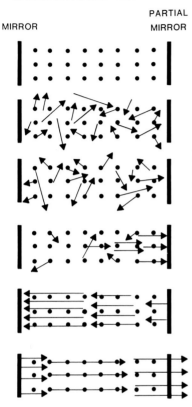

FIG 2–7.
Events in a laser resonator consist of excitation of an active medium. The randomly generated spontaneously emitted photons are fed back through the gain medium in an optical cavity with a partially transmitting mirror output to produce a directional laser beam.

LASER DEVICES

Argon Ion Lasers

The argon ion laser has been used extensively for medical procedures and is a well-developed laser system. It operates on a CW basis and is capable of average powers up to approximately 20 W. The laser emits radiation at a variety of wavelengths, but the wavelengths most commonly selected for medical use are in the blue-green spectral region at 488 to 514 nm. The population inversion in argon gas is produced by passing a very high electric discharge current through the gas. Figure 2–8 shows the energy level diagram for producing a population inversion in electronic states of argon ion. In this case, the discharge in the argon gas produces high-energy electrons that collide with argon atoms to excite and ionize the atom. Note that the upper laser level requires 35 eV of energy to produce the upper laser level in the singly charged argon ion. This upper level radiates to a lower energy level of argon ion with the emission of a photon at 514 nm, which has an energy of only 2.5 eV. Therefore, the ultimate theoretical efficiency of this laser device is 2.5/35 ×

100% or 7%, but in reality the overall efficiency is much less than this because of the low probability of electron impact producing the upper state and because of low optical extraction efficiency. In practice, the overall efficiency of an argon ion laser is only about 0.1%, which means that the power supply has to produce 20 kW of power to generate 20 W of green laser light.

The lower laser level in the argon ion transition radiates spontaneously away in the vacuum ultraviolet wavelength region. This is typical of multilevel visible and ultraviolet laser transitions. To create a population inversion between electronic energy levels, the laser transition must be of lower energy than the transition from the lower level to its next lower energy state. This condition requires that the rate of energy loss by collision or radiation be proportional to the magnitude of energy transition difference between the two levels. Therefore, visible and ultraviolet lasers are inherently much more inefficient converters of electrical to light energy, since they operate on a multiple-level transition scheme. Since 99.9% of the 20 kW of electrical power ends up as heat in the laser gain medium, this thermal energy must be removed or the high temperatures will rapidly destroy the laser tube. The need to remove large quantities of heat adds significant cooling requirements, which further complicate laser design.

The blue-green light of the argon ion laser is primarily absorbed by chromogens and hemoglobin and it penetrates tissue to a greater extent than ultraviolet and far-infrared light. The absorption of focused high-power argon radiation leads to heating of the irradiated area. If chromophores are present, argon laser energy is useful for applications that require selective localized heating of tissue. However, the excessive penetration into most tissue with the concomitant lateral scattering and large heat-affected zone preclude CW irra-

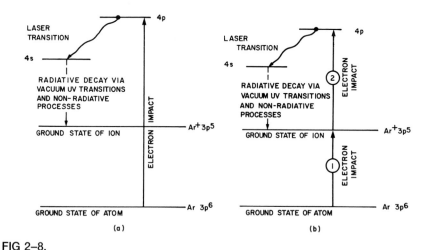

FIG 2–8.
Energy level diagram for a singly ionized argon (Ar) laser. There are two electron excitation mechanisms: **A,** a single excitation from the ground level of Ar to the upper level of Ar$^+$; and **B,** a two-step electron excitation process. *UV* indicates ultraviolet; *s* and *p* are spectroscopic designators for orbits of the excited electrons.

diation using this wavelength for controlled ablation applications. In fact, the use of CW argon laser for angioplasty has been hindered by the lack of control of ablation and by deep heating of the vessel wall.[11] Considerable improvement in the use of this laser for angioplasty has been achieved by converting the laser energy into heat at a metal cap and using the laser in essence as an electrocautery device to minimize the depth of heat penetration into the blood vessel wall.[12] Since the visible wavelength is readily transmitted by glass optical fibers, this laser energy can easily be delivered in medical procedures.

The CO_2 Laser

The CO_2 is an infrared laser operating on a molecular vibrational energy transition and lases at 10.6 μm. The laser can be operated at high power levels on a CW basis, on a radio frequency (RF) excited basis, and as a high peak power pulsed transversely excited (TEA) laser. Although each type of operation mentioned still produces a laser beam at 10.6 μm, the nature of the laser device is different, and the beam of 10.6-μm radiation from each type of CO_2 laser device can produce substantially different effects on tissue, although they all go by the name CO_2 laser.

The active medium in the CO_2 laser is CO_2, but additions of nitrogen (N_2) and He are important for its operation. Figure 2–9 shows the energy diagram for the laser transition. Note that for an infrared laser it is easier to operate at energy levels close to the ground level, providing for a more favorable efficiency. In this laser, an electric discharge is established in the gas mixture and the N_2 is raised to an excited vibrational level by collisions with electrons in the discharge. Because the N_2 molecule is symmetric and has no permanent dipole, it does not lose the excited vibrational energy by radiation; in effect it is trapped in a metastable state and transfers its excess energy in a collision with a CO_2 ground-state molecule, which rises to an excited vibrational level of CO_2 in close energy resonance with the excited N_2 molecule. The CO_2 molecule, however, does have a dipole-allowed radiation transition at 10.6 μm; therefore, once the energy deposited in N_2 from the electric discharge is transferred from excited N_2 to CO_2, laser action can occur and the intermediate CO_2 energy levels are rapidly depopulated by radiation and collisions with He. The He gas also rapidly removes heat from the system so that the lower levels in the CO_2 transition do not become heavily populated. The CO_2 laser can be very efficient, on the order of 10%.

It is much easier to produce a population inversion between vibrational-rotational levels than electronic levels. However, the limitation of this argument is that the pump source, which in this case is an electrical discharge, tends to decompose molecular species, which limits the utility of the laser gain medium unless the gas mixture is continually replaced. For the CO_2 laser, the discharge dissociates the CO_2 molecule, producing CO and O_2, which are detrimental to laser action. It is the inability of the gain medium to regenerate itself that limits the types of practical laser devices that have been demonstrated for molecular infrared lasers.

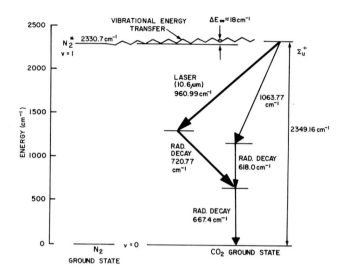

FIG 2–9.
Energy level diagram showing the transfer of energy from vibrationally excited metastable nitrogen (N_2^*) to the upper level of vibronically excited carbon dioxide (CO_2), which produces lasing at 10.6 μm. v indicates vibrational quantum number; RAD, radiative; $\Delta E\infty$, energy separation between metastable N_2^* and the upper laser level state of CO_2; Σ_u^+, spectroscopic symbol for energy level of CO_2.

The CO_2 laser wavelength is strongly absorbed by water vapor, and since most tissue has a large water content, the penetration depth of this wavelength is small, and only local superficial heating is produced, in contrast to the visible and near-infrared wavelengths. This wavelength is good for local heating, microsurgery, and surface coagulation. However, the particular procedures for this laser wavelength should be carefully evaluated for the choice of laser beam delivery (i.e., pulsed vs. CW) and the peak power of the pulsed laser application. Although the CO_2 laser has found a wide acceptance for use in medical procedures, its utility is limited by the lack of availability of suitable flexible fiberoptic delivery; it is usually delivered by means of awkward, flexible, articulated arms or short, hollow waveguide tubes. The CO_2 has been used for intraoperative coronary laser angioplasty, but the laser energy has had to be delivered through a short, hollow, metal waveguide.[13] The use of CW or RF excited CO_2 lasers, which are compact, simple devices, may not be as appropriate for cardiovascular surgery as use of a higher-power pulsed TEA CO_2 laser, especially if calcified material needs to be removed without extensive heat deposition into surrounding tissue.

Solid-State Lasers: The Nd:YAG

This laser is an example of a solid-state laser gain medium instead of the gaseous lasers discussed before. Solid-state lasers are optically pumped either

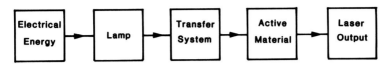

FIG 2–10.
General scheme of an optically pumped laser system. Each box is coupled with a certain energy transfer efficiency. The total laser efficiency is the product of the individual efficiencies.

by incoherent broad spectral radiation produced by a flashlamp or by another laser. Figure 2–10 shows the method of optical pumping. Electrical energy is passed through a gas discharge flashlamp, producing excited species that radiate the excited energy by spontaneous emission. A solid laser rod intercepts some of the randomly emitted flashlamp radiation, and a portion of the broad spectral output is absorbed into an excited energy state. Figure 2–11 shows the energy level diagram for the Nd:YAG laser. Excited levels of Nd are produced when radiation in only the 0.73- and 0.8-μm wavelength regions are absorbed from the flashlamp. Since only a portion of the laser rod is pumped by the flashlamp and only a fraction of the output of the flashlamp is emitted in the appropriate wavelength regions, the efficiency of the laser is only about 1% overall. The Nd:YAG laser is a four-level laser transition, which facilitates maintaining a population inversion. This laser can be run either CW or pulsed. One advantage of a solid-state laser gain medium is that more active species for the upper laser population can be produced than in a gas or liquid per unit volume of the gain region, owing to the increased density in a solid matrix. Additionally, the upper excited laser state can be stored before the stimulated emission process is initiated, and the energy can be released as short

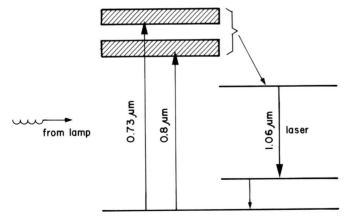

FIG 2–11.
Simplified level schematic for neodymium: YAG laser transition. Note the upper starting laser levels are produced by absorption of narrow bands in the 0.7- to 0.8-μm region from the broad spectral output of the flashlamp.

intense optical pulses by an optical feedback mechanism. This technique, called "Q-switching" the laser produces high-peak-power pulses in the range of 10 nsec and less from a pulsed Nd:YAG laser. These high-power Q-switched pulses can be used for nonlinear second harmonic generation in a suitable crystal host to convert substantial fractions (40% to 50%) of the 1.06-μm radiation into the green at 0.532 μm. Additional frequency conversion to produce 0.352 and 0.266 μm can be done but with decreasing efficiency. The efficient generation of the various harmonics of the Nd:YAG laser is peak-power dependent; therefore, the harmonics are best produced with short pulses at high peak power produced by a Q-switched laser.

The disadvantage of solid-state lasers, as in most lasers, is still the low laser efficiency, about 1%; the rest of the pump energy is rapidly degraded into heat in the solid host. Heat can damage the expensive laser rod and also cause the laser beam to be distorted in passage through the laser gain medium if a temperature gradient exists. Other types of optically pumped solid-state lasers are the alexandrite laser, which lases at 0.760 μm, the ruby laser at 0.68 μm, and the erbium (Er)–YAG and Er:YLF lasers, which radiate near 3.0 μm.

The 1.06-μm radiation of the Nd:YAG laser is readily transmitted through silica fiberoptics. This laser can operate at high average powers CW and high peak powers for pulsed applications, and its output can be converted to shorter wavelengths. This makes this laser a very versatile tool. The 1.06-μm radiation has deep penetration into tissue, causing heat generation beyond the surface of irradiation, as used for coagulation and tumor necrosis. To localize the heating produced by CW laser irradiation at 1.06 μm, sapphire tips have been used. As with the argon laser probe with a metal cap at the end of the fiberoptic, this turns the laser into a heating probe similar to an electrocautery device. Microablation using the shorter-wavelength harmonics of Nd:YAG is possible but suffers from the decreased laser efficiency when the frequency is changed and from difficulty in transmitting high-peak-power pulses through fiberoptics even though the fibers are transparent to these wavelengths. Since high-peak-power pulses are necessary to produce the other wavelengths, this may present a problem for efficient fiber delivery.

The Er:YAG laser is of considerable interest for microsurgical applications because the strong water absorption at 3.0 μm makes this laser similar to the CO_2 laser for small penetration into tissue. Although this laser is not as well developed or as versatile as the CO_2 laser, it does have efficient fiberoptic transmission, which the CO_2 laser lacks. However, other aspects of fluoride infrared fibers, such as low flexibility, brittleness, and poor strength, make them less applicable than plastic or silica fibers. For many medical procedures, if one cannot get the laser radiation conveniently to the target, in most cases by fiberoptics, then the laser will have limited use.

Dye Lasers

Dye lasers are another example of an optically pumped laser system. Either a flashlamp or another laser is used to pump the liquid dye solution.

Depending on the dye chosen, laser emission can be obtained in a particular portion of the wavelength spectrum from the near ultraviolet through the near infrared. These lasers can be operated at either a CW or a pulsed mode. The dye laser is very useful as a general-purpose laser to determine the optimum wavelength for a medical procedure. However, these laser systems are complicated since the dye must be circulated through a chamber, since dye lifetime is rather short, and since the dye solution must be replaced regularly. As discussed previously, except for pigments that selectively absorb visible light, strong absorption by tissue occurs in either the infrared or the ultraviolet, where dye lasers do not operate efficiently.

Excimer Lasers

The excimer gas laser is one of the few lasers that operate directly in the ultraviolet spectral region, and it only operates in a pulsed mode of operation (i.e., it does not operate CW). The word *excimer* stands for excited dimer, and there are a variety of excimer lasers that operate in regions of the ultraviolet from 0.193 to 0.351 μm. The laser is produced by a high-voltage, transverse-pulsed electric discharge on a high-pressure gas mixture containing several atmospheres of an inert gas, such as He, Ne, or argon, and several percent of another inert gas, such as Xe or krypton (Kr), and a much smaller percentage, around 0.1%, of a halogen compound such as hydrogen chloride or fluorine (F_2). The excimers, or rare-gas halide lasers, are unusual lasers as they are a two-level energy system and the gas is very good at regenerating itself between pulses to the original starting species, allowing for long sealed operation, in particular for the Cl lasers. The electric discharge ionizes and causes electronic excitation of the minor inert gas species, such as Xe, in the discharge. At the same time, the electrons in the discharge produce negative halogen ions, such as Cl^-. The Xe + ion is strongly attracted to the negative halogen ion to produce an ionically bound molecule in an excited state (i.e., XeCl), which is similar in electronic structure to salts such as sodium chloride. When this excimer molecule radiates, it goes to the lower ground level of XeCl, which is covalently bonded very weakly, as the Xe atom has returned to its inert gas electronic configuration. This lower energy state of the XeCl molecule rapidly separates to the individual atoms. Therefore, the lower laser molecular level is lost as soon as it is formed, and there is very little population in this level to stop laser action.

Excimer lasing actions from ArF at 0.193 μm, KrCl at 0.222 μm, XeCl at 0.308 μm, and XeF at 0.351 μm are examples of a class of intense pulsed laser sources of ultraviolet radiation. Since these lasers are relatively new devices, their use in the medical field is rather recent. The output pulse width obtainable from these devices ranges from under 10 nsec to several hundred. Descriptions of the excimer laser kinetics and laser design are found in the literature.[14, 15]

The advantage of the excimer laser for medical applications is the strong absorption by tissue in the ultraviolet range, which minimizes penetration heating and provides for microsurgical procedures. The ArF laser, at 0.193 μm, has the strongest absorption but has been used mostly for corneal applications, since this wavelength is difficult to transmit through present fiberoptics. The XeCl laser and the XeF laser are readily transmitted through high-purity silica-based fiberoptics, provided the pulse width of the laser is long enough to keep the power density on the fiber below its destruction level. Precise ablation of calcified and fatty plaque using long-pulse 0.308-μm radiation through a fiber-optic has been demonstrated.[10] At present, the XeCl laser is the most appropriate laser source for pulsed ultraviolet angioplasty since it is (1) a very efficient laser device (1% to 4%), (2) has the most benign long-lived gas mixture of all the excimer lasers, and (3) is readily transmitted through fiberoptics when operated at pulse widths greater than 100 nsec.

For microsurgical applications there is a requirement for strong absorption by the laser wavelength to limit the ablation area and volume per pulse. Either infrared or ultraviolet wavelengths are needed for tissues that do not possess a strong visible chromophore or pigment. In the infrared, the CO_2 laser is hampered by the lack of an adequate fiberoptic delivery system, and the newer Er:YAG and Er:YLF lasers need more development for both the laser and the fiberoptic delivery system, but there is promise that these engineering issues may be solved. The excimer lasers have not been as extensively refined for use in the medical environment, but there is no major engineering problem to prevent achievement of a proper medical design. Fiberoptic delivery is possible for long–pulse-width XeCl and XeF laser radiation at 0.308 and 0.351 μm. Besides proper system engineering, questions regarding possible mutagenic effects of the ultraviolet wavelength have to be addressed. Adequate fiberoptic delivery at the shorter ultraviolet wavelengths, such as 0.193 and 0.248 μm, have yet to be demonstrated satisfactorily. The main promise for the use of ultraviolet wavelengths is the high efficiency for ablation of most materials owing to the direct photochemical molecular dissociation mechanism[16] vs. rapid heating, as is the mechansim for infrared ablation. In addition, the ultraviolet does not require a water absorption mechanism to transfer the light energy to the tissue; therefore, it is possible to pass some ultraviolet wavelengths through fluid media, such as saline solution, with limited attenuation. Obviously, further work is necessary to study the differences between ablation from the two wavelength regions in the ultraviolet and infrared.

LASER-TISSUE INTERACTION

The fundamentals of how laser light is produced by the laser device have been presented, but the physician is dealing with the effects of that laser radiation on tissue. To understand tissue response to laser light radiation, several optical variables must be specified. These are the irradiance level, the energy fluence, and the exposure time, which provide the total light energy dosage. Therefore, these variables of laser light must always be specified: (1) the energy delivered per unit of time, (2) the spot size of the area irradiated, and (3) the time of irradiation and, if pulsed laser is used, the duration of the laser pulse. There are two types of laser light power designations, average power and peak power when a pulsed laser is used. Average power is the energy delivered per unit of time, whereas peak power is the energy contained in a single laser pulse divided by its pulse width. The pulse width is typically measured using a fast photodetection-oscilloscope combination, and for a symmetric pulse shape the width is defined as the width at half the maximum of the peak of the pulse. The average power delivered by a pulsed laser is the total energy delivered per unit of time, which equals the number of pulses per second from the laser times the individual pulse energy. These two forms of average power level, one for a pulsed laser and the other for a CW laser, usually produce distinctly different effects on tissue even when the total energy dosage is the same and the wavelength is the same. Designating average power without knowing the other characteristics of the laser, especially if used in a pulsed manner, is insufficient for understanding the procedure. In all cases, the irradiance or power per unit area is the important characteristic for understanding a laser procedure. For example, if a pulsed laser produces pulses with energy of 100 mJ at 100 pulses per second with a 10-nsec pulse duration in a 1-sq cm spot size, its average power density is 100 mJ times 100 pulses per second per square centimeter or 10 W/sq cm average power, but the peak power is 100 mJ $\div$ 10 $\times$ 10^{-9} sec/sq cm, or 10 megawatts/sq cm. For pulsed lasers, both the average as well as peak power density or irradiance values are important. For CW lasers, the irradiance is equal to the laser power output from the laser divided by the laser beam cross section at the tissue site, and its unit is watts per square centimeter.

The primary uniqueness of energy in the form of laser light is the ability to concentrate the light energy both spatially as well as temporally to cause very high levels of local energy deposition, which cannot be easily achieved using other sources or forms of energy. The energy fluence is the energy per pulse divided by the beam spot area and is expressed in joules per square centimeter. For a CW laser the energy fluence is given by the laser output power in watts times the exposure time in seconds divided by the area irradiated.

Once these parameters of the laser light are measured, the next important effect is absorption and scattering of the light energy by the tissue, which is typically wavelength dependent. The three basic mechanisms of absorption of laser light are shown in Figure 2–12. The most common for CW lasers or pulsed lasers in the visible and infrared is the conversion of the absorbed photons into heat or thermal motion of the molecules that compose tissue. As heat is deposited into an irradiated area, there is thermal conduction by the tissue to its surrounding area. To minimize the lateral spread of this heat conduction, either a pulsed laser with a pulse duration shorter than the characteristic thermal conduction time of the tissue is used or a very small area is irradiated. As the absorbed laser energy is converted into heat, the tempera-

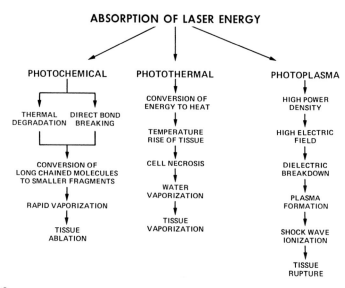

FIG 2–12.
Schematic of three types of energy deposition mechanisms in tissue following absorption of laser energy.

ture of the tissue rises, causing cell necrosis. The temperature of the tissue continues to rise until it reaches the level where water vaporization occurs, and then the temperature rises until tissue vaporization occurs. This thermal absorption process occurs with both CW and pulsed laser sources when the pulse duration is greater than the thermal diffusion time for the tissue or the energy per pulse is below ablation threshold.

The other two absorption mechanisms in medical applications are predominantly produced by high-peak-power pulsed laser sources. The photoplasma mechanism is somewhat independent of laser wavelength and can occur in materials normally transparent to the laser wavelength at low power levels. Very high-peak-power laser radiation produces a very intense local electric field, causing dielectric breakdown of material and heating of liberated electrons, which avalanche to produce a local plasma. The sudden expansion of vaporized material produces a shock wave, causing localized rupture of the tissue. This process is used in ophthalmology where the laser beam can be focused into the eye. At the focal spot, the power density is high enough to produce tissue ablation by means of dielectric breakdown. This mechanism works on materials that are normally transparent to the laser wavelength at low intensity; this mechanism can also destroy optics and solid laser rods if any high laser power densities are incident on the optical elements. The third mechanism only pertains to short-pulse ultraviolet wavelengths and is called photochemical ablation. The energy of an ultraviolet photon if absorbed by a molecule can rupture the molecular bonds directly, causing a change of a large molecule to smaller fragment molecules, which then leave the substrate in a rapid expansion. This is a very efficient tissue ablation mechanism and produces clean incisions with minimal thermal heat retention in the nonirradiated tissue when short-pulsed ultraviolet laser sources are used (10 to 300 nsec). This process requires a strong absorption of the laser wavelength by the tissue in the ultraviolet, and for pulsed ultraviolet sources, multiphoton processes may occur as well as single photon absorption for the photochemical bond-breaking mechanism.

Figure 2–13 is a general material processing graph[17] for pulsed lasers. The effects of laser light at a given wavelength can produce different effects depending on the power density and pulse duration used. The aspect of absorption depth is not contained in this graph. Note that if a pulse of laser energy is applied over a long time, then that laser pulse will have a lower power density than the same energy delivered in a shorter pulse duration to the same spot size. To melt a material for welding, one needs to heat the material to a certain depth and not have it cool too rapidly or have the material rapidly vaporize. One can see that this process requires the energy to be delivered over a longer period or at lower power densities than for vaporization. If the power density level is low, heating without vaporization occurs because the absorbed heat is conducted away too rapidly to allow the material temperature to reach its vaporization level. Therefore, for efficient welding of tissue, the appropriate wavelength for the desired penetration depth is used, and the power density must be in a narrow region to prevent excess vaporization. If

PULSED LASER MATERIAL PROCESSING

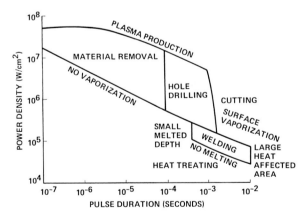

FIG 2–13.
Generalized schematic of laser power density and pulse duration suitable for material processing applications. This schematic will vary with target material and laser wavelength. (From Ready JF: *Industrial Application of Lasers.* New York, Academic Press, 1978. Reproduced by permission.)

vaporization for material removal is required, the laser energy must be delivered at a higher power density. If the power density exceeds dielectric breakdown level, plasma production occurs. The control of the value of power density is achieved by varying the pulse duration of the laser, and the energy density is controlled by changing the area of the spot size, as shown in Figure 2–14. The smaller the spot size the higher the power density. Note that the control of spot size using a focusing lens strongly depends on the focal length of the lens and position of the lens from the tissue surface.

The high power densities produced by laser radiation on small areas provide very localized photobiologic effects on tissue, and there is a specific minimum energy dosage required to effect tissue change on a given volume of tissue. If the laser radiation is just converted into thermal energy and subsequent heating of the tissue, the biologic effects of heat are nonspecific to the laser wavelength. The choice of laser wavelength just determines the depth of penetration of the energy deposition and extent of scattering into the tissue. The use of short pulses temporarily to concentrate the laser power density further can yield substantially different biologic effects on tissue. The wavelength in the case of the photoablation mechanism needs to be in the ultraviolet.

In conclusion, when performing a laser procedure it is best to think of the laser device as only an optical power generator and carefully consider the combination of laser wavelength, irradiance, and energy fluence used. The same type of laser, if operated in a different output mode, can cause considerably different tissue effects even though the wavelength is the same. It is

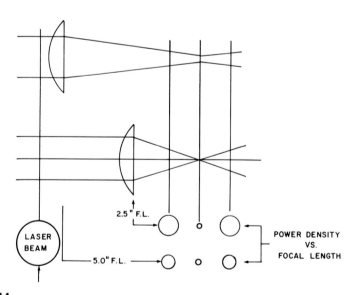

FIG 2–14.
Power density vs. focal length *(F.L.)* for a focused laser beam showing the relationship between laser spot size and power density with distance from the lens.

important to understand the nature of the interaction of the light energy with the tissue for each procedure. The necessity for the large size of the laser device with its associated heat exchangers and power supplies is due to the inefficiency of converting electric energy into the precise controlled energy in the form of a collimated, coherent laser beam. For certain medical procedures the therapeutic effect of this form of energy more than compensates for the cost and complexity of medical laser devices.

REFERENCES

1. Maiman TH: Stimulated optical radiation in ruby. *Nature* 1960; 187:493–494.
2. Javan A, Bennett WR Jr, Herroit DQ: Population inversion and continuous optical laser oscillation in a gaseous discharge containing a He-Ne mixture. *Phys Rev Lett* 1961; 6:106–110.
3. Bridges WB: Laser oscillation in singly ionized argon in the visible spectrum. *Appl Phys Lett* 1964; 4:128–130.
4. Bell WE: Visible laser transitions in Hg^+. *Appl Phys Lett* 1964; 4:34–35.
5. Patel CKN: Continuous wave laser action on vibrational-rotational transitions of CO_2. *Phys Rev* 1964; 136:A1187–A1193.
6. Burham R, Harris NW, Djeu N: Xenon fluoride laser excitation by transverse electric discharge. *Appl Phys Lett* 1976; 28:86–87
7. Wang CP, Mirels H, Sutton DG, et al: Fast-discharge-initiated XeF laser. *Appl Phys Lett* 1976; 28:236–238.
8. Laudenslager JB, Pacala TJ, Wittig C: Electric discharge pumped nitrogen ion laser. *Appl Phys Lett* 1976; 29:580–582.
9. Fuller TA: Fundamentals of lasers in surgery and medicine, in Dixon JA (ed): *Surgical Application of Lasers*. Chicago, Year Book Medical Publishers, 1983, pp 11–28.
10. Forrester JS, Litvack F, Grundfest WS: Laser angioplasty and cardiovascular disease. *Am J Cardiol* 1986; 57:990–992.
11. Ginsburg R, Wexler L, Mitchell RS, et al: Percutaneous transluminal laser angioplasty for treatment of peripheral vascular disease: Clinical experience with 16 patients. *Radiology* 1985; 156:619–624.
12. Sanborn TA, Faxon DP, Haudenschild CC, et al: Experimental angioplasty: Circumferential distribution of laser thermal energy with a laser probe. *J Am Coll Cardiol* 1985; 5:934–938.
13. Livesay JJ, Leachman DR, Hogan PJ, et al: Preliminary report on laser coronary endarterectomy in patients, abstracted. *Circulation* 1985; 72(suppl 3):III–302.
14. Brau CA: Rare gas halogen excimers, in Rhodes CK (ed): *Excimer Lasers*. New York, Springer-Verlag New York, 1979.
15. Laudenslager JB: Ion-molecule processes in lasers, Ausloos P (ed): *Kinetics of Ion-Molecule Reactions*. New York, Plenum Publishing Corp, 1978.
16. Srinivasan R, Leigh WJ: Ablative photodecomposition action of far-ultraviolet (193 μm) laser radiation on poly (ethylene/terephthalate) films. *J Am Chem Soc* 1985; 150:220–226.
17. Ready JF: *Industrial Application of Lasers*. New York, Academic Press, 1978, p 356.

3

Laser-Tissue Interactions: Considerations for Cardiovascular Applications*

Warren S. Grundfest, M.D.

Frank I. Litvack, M.D.

D. Lynn Doyle, M.D., F.R.C.S.(C.)

James S. Forrester, M.D.

The objectives of this chapter are to review laser-tissue interactions as functions of type of laser, components of tissue, and mode of energy delivery. Though there are many types of lasers, the one common denominator is their ability to deliver intense, monochromatic radiation to a small area of tissue. The incident laser energy may be reflected with minimal effect on the tissue. The energy may be absorbed, and, depending on the wavelength, the depth of penetration, and the absorption characteristics of the tissue, the incident energy may be converted to heat, may be emitted as fluorescence, or may directly photoactivate chemical bonds. At very high intensities (>1 megawatt), the laser energy forms an expanding "plasma" in the tissue and generates an explosive shock wave. This "explosion" may lead to tissue removal. Each of these processes leads to fundamentally different outcomes.

*This experimental work is supported in part by the Imperial Grand Sweepstakes, the Grand Sweepstakes, and the Medallion Funds of Cedars-Sinai Medical Center. This work is also supported in part by Specialized Centers of Research in Ischemic Heart Disease of the National Heart, Lung, and Blood Institute grant #HL-17651. Doctors Grundfest and Litvack are recipients of NHLBI clinical awards #HL-01522 and #HL-01381 respectively.

The choice of laser depends on the application. Results of the laser-tissue interaction can be predicted if the following information is known:

1. The wavelength of the laser energy.
2. The time span and intensity of the delivered light.
3. Absorption characteristics of the tissue. If the energy is reflected there will be little effect; if the energy is absorbed at the tissue surface only those cells irradiated may be affected. However, if the light scatters and penetrates deeply into the tissue, the effects of this energy may occur at some site distant from the point of irradiation.

Attempts to produce mathematical models of the laser-tissue interaction are complicated by the great heterogenicity of tissue and the changes that occur during irradiation. Any model must account for optical scattering, absorption, and reflection. These parameters change during the irradiation, making all but the simplest models very complex and difficult to use. When additional factors such as tissue heterogenicity, thickness, and boundary layers are considered, accurate modeling with differential equations becomes mathematically complex and difficult, if not impossible, to solve.

TYPES OF LASER-TISSUE INTERACTIONS

Physical Processes

The choice of laser radiation depends on the desired outcome of the absorption and transmission of the energy. Energy that is not absorbed at the surface of the tissue can be scattered and absorbed at areas remote from the site of irradiation. The effect of the scattered energy depends on the depth of penetration of energy and the presence of absorbing molecules (chromophores). If the energy is delivered in short, intense pulses, or if boiling and ejection of material occur, acoustic transients can be set up within tissue, causing cavitation. Cavitation can lead to loss of tissue architecture. A "photoplasma" explosion can vaporize tissue and cause disruption in the surrounding zone adjacent to the explosion.

Thermal Process

When the absorbed energy is dissipated primarily as heat, tissue changes occur along a predictable continuum as the heat increases. Tissue welding by lasers occurs at relatively low temperatures. Heating of the tissue from 43 to 50° C may allow for the uncoiling and annealing of collagen helices so that apposed tissue edges may be fused by reforming covalent bonds. As the tissue temperature increases, between 50 and 60° C, irreversible protein denaturation and subsequent cell death occur.[1] Beyond 60° C, cell death is inevitable. As temperatures reach 90 to 100° C, the underlying collagen and elastin structures begin to degrade. At temperatures greater than 100° C, melting, boiling, ablation, and pyrolysis occur, resulting in tissue ablation. Ablation temperatures for calcified tissues may exceed 500° C.

When laser energy is converted to heat in the tissues, thermal diffusion begins. Diffusion of heat through the tissue depends on the thermal properties of the irradiated material. Vascular tissue tends to have thermal diffusion constants in a range of 1 to 10 μ/sec.[2] Pulses longer than several microseconds will allow thermal energy to diffuse over 10 to 100 μm in a few milliseconds. Pulses in the millisecond range are sufficiently long to allow for heat generated to diffuse between 100 and 1,000 μm away from the zone of irradiation. The thermal relaxation (cooling) phenomenon is influenced by (1) the thermal coefficient of the tissue, (2) the properties of the surrounding tissue or fluids, and (3) the temperature differential between the irradiated and nonirradiated tissue.[3]

Photochemical Processes

Photochemical change can occur as a result of direct excitation of electronic bonds by the laser energy and is one of the proposed mechanisms of action of pulsed, ultraviolet lasers. Electronic excitation by laser is not 100% efficient; therefore, heat is also generated during this process. The physical chemistry of pulsed tissue ablation is as yet not well defined. Two potential mechanisms appear to operate.[4] At shorter wavelengths, tissue components, proteins, and lipids absorb photons and become electronically excited. This "photoexcitation" leads to rupture of molecular bonds and formation of molecular fragments. These molecular fragments then undergo a process known as photochemical desorption and are ejected from the irradiated surface in less than 1 μ/sec. The ejected fragments carry with them much of the energy that was initially deposited within the tissue to generate the fragments. This electronic excitation occurs before conversion to heat or thermal diffusion occurs. A second possible mechanism to explain this phenomenon is very high-speed, localized absorption, which leads to formation of a very small area of vaporized photoproducts. These products expand rapidly away from the tissue surface, again carrying away the incident energy. The result of optimal pulsed ultraviolet ablation is tissue removal with minimal thermal damage to adjacent structures.

Fluorescent Phenomena

Fluorescence occurs when photons of light are absorbed by tissue and reemitted at a longer wavelength. This rapidly occurring process (nanoseconds or less) is strongly affected by the electronic bond structure and the chemical composition of the irradiated matter. Fluorescence can be used to detect and monitor specific compounds that occur naturally or that have been added to the system. A particular wavelength fluorescence must be distinguished from the baseline autofluorescence that occurs in tissue. This can be done using various filters after identifying the specific wavelengths of the emitted (fluorescent) light. To date this work has primarily focused on photodetection of hematoporphyrin derivatives,[5, 6] tetracycline,[7] and carotenoids.[8]

Laser-induced fluorescence results when a portion of the laser light is absorbed and reradiated. Given the high intensity and monochromaticity of the laser beam, the reradiated light can be of sufficient intensity to permit detection and analysis. The returning fluorescent light pattern can act as a fingerprint for identification of certain compounds. Analysis of the fluorescent pattern is now under study as a means of differentiating normal from atherosclerotic tissue.[9, 10] This would permit target-specific laser angioplasty. Preliminary results are encouraging; however, the laser-induced fluorescence is so sensitive to chemical changes that irradiated or ablated tissue may give different signals than normal or atherosclerotic tissue.

QUANTITATION OF THE LASER-TISSUE INTERACTION

Our group uses high-speed filming, quantitative ocular micrometry, and tissue thermal analysis to characterize and quantitate the changes that occur during laser-tissue interactions. High-speed filming allows us to slow down events that happen too rapidly to be seen with the naked eye. Figure 3–1 displays a schematic of the high-speed filming apparatus. This arrangement permits the study of laser energy delivered either through a fiberoptic waveguide or directly from the ouput mirror to a tissue specimen mounted on a platform or immersed in fluid, usually saline solution. Quantitative ocular micrometry of histologic sections of irradiated tissue permits quantitation of the depth and width of the lesions created by the laser-tissue interaction. Temporal and spatial analysis of the thermal gradients generated at the tissue interface defines the role of tissue heating in the ablative process. These observations are made using an infrared thermal camera (AGA 782) (Fig 3–2). This camera

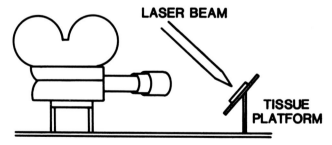

FIG 3–1.
Schematic diagram of the experimental apparatus for high-speed film analysis. The laser beam is carried either by a fiberoptic waveguide or directly from the output mirror and is aimed at the tissue platform containing atherosclerotic human aorta. The film or video moves at 500 to 6,000 frames per second, giving an expansion of time from 20:1 to 500:1.

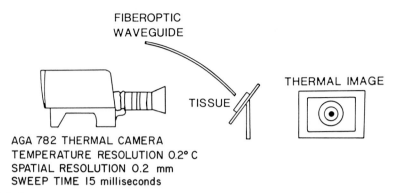

AGA 782 THERMAL CAMERA
TEMPERATURE RESOLUTION 0.2° C
SPATIAL RESOLUTION 0.2 mm
SWEEP TIME 15 milliseconds

FIG 3–2.
To achieve a thermal map or picture of the heat generated, we use a thermal digital camera (AGA 782). This has a temperature resolution of 0.2° C, a spatial resolution of 0.2 mm, and a sweep time of 15 msec. The thermal camera is aimed at the target tissue, in vitro or in vivo, and real-time images are displayed on a monitor and stored on videotape. Selected frames are then transferred to a computer, where detailed analysis of the thermal image at any given time can be performed.

allows for continuous high-resolution recordings of the heat generated at the tissue surface during the laser-tissue interaction. With the use of appropriate filters and standards, very accurate temperature measurements can be made. In addition, zones of temperature changes can be recorded and followed.

Using this methodology, we have observed that tissue responds to heating with a slight volume expansion. As heating proceeds above 50° C, protein denaturation occurs. Time exposure is critical since exposures of less than a microsecond may not result in cell death, whereas exposures of greater than a millisecond usually produce irreversible protein denaturation. As temperatures rise above 60° C, extracellular proteins and collagen fibers begin to denature. Such loss of structure is seen histologically as coagulation injury or hypereosinophilia of the tissue. As heating proceeds beyond 100° C, water begins to boil, leaving behind vacuoles within the remaining proteinaceous structure of the coagulated tissue. Vacuoles are telltale signs of temperatures in excess of 100° C. As temperatures rise above 125° C, complete oxidation of the protein and lipids occurs, leaving behind carbon particles. This carbonization or charring of the tissue surface indicates relatively high temperature processes. Explosive vaporization of water or transmission of shock waves induced by pulsed lasers is evidenced by development of vacuoles and loss of tissue architecture. Shock wave injury can be quite prominent and independent of thermal injury.

Continuous-Wave Laser-Tissue Interactions

We have performed a series of high-speed camera observations using continuous-wave neodymium:yttrium-aluminum-garnet (Nd:YAG), continuous-wave argon ion, and continuous-wave ultraviolet laser sources. High-speed filming of these processes is most informative (Plate 1). The first observation is that the tissue blanches as the chromophores are bleached. Second, the tissue begins to melt, and a molten pool of material appears immediately under the area of irradiation. Surrounding this molten pool, a small, raised crater rim develops and boiling begins. As heating continues, steam can be seen rising from the tissue surface. This is sometimes accompanied by ejection of relatively large particles. As the temperature deep to the tissue surface rises, explosive ejection of tissue fragments promptly follows. As all of the molten material evaporates, pyrolysis of the tissue occurs. Concentric zones of thermal injury develop and continue to expand as the ablative process continues. Deep to the crater surface, boiling continues. During this phase of ablation, material deep to the crater flows into the area being directly ablated. This material undergoes intense laser irradiation and is usually carbonized rapidly. The zone of thermal injury expands radially outward and beneath the tissue surface, and molten material from lateral heating continues to flow into the crater. In summary, continuous-wave lasers ablate tissue by a series of overlapping phases. Tissue first blanches due to protein denaturation and loss of hydration, then melts. As heating continues, boiling ensues, followed by pyrolysis and carbonization of the tissue concomitant with lateral thermal injury.

Pulsed Ultraviolet Laser-Tissue Interactions

Pulsed ultraviolet lasers, in particular those operating at wavelengths less than 337 nm, produce tissue ablation through a different process. High-speed film observations made during irradiation of atherosclerotic aortic tissue with a 308-nm excimer laser or with a pulsed frequency-tripled Nd:YAG laser at 266 nm have shown that the ablative process occurs with each pulse. These laser pulses range from 7 to 200 nanoseconds (nsec). Such intense pulses of energy have profoundly different effects on the tissue compared with those seen with the continuous-wave irradiation. The first three to four pulses appear to have little impact on the tissue, then ablation begins with each pulse. No lateral thermal effects are seen if the area is irradiated at or above ablation threshold limits. As irradiation proceeds, the ablated area corresponds precisely to the area irradiated at or above threshold limits (Plate 2).

Thermal injury can occur with pulsed lasers either at high repetition rates, in which there is insufficient time to allow for thermal relaxation of the tissue, or by irradiation at subthreshold levels. High repetition rates also tend to produce significant zones of blast injury. Quantitative ocular micrometry can quantify the extent of histologically observable laser-induced damage. This technique can also be used to compare and contrast the effects of different lasers on vascular tissue. As demonstrated in Plate 3, attempts to produce a 2-mm–deep zone of ablation can have widely variable results depending on the choice of laser. Predictable ablation is a critical factor in developing a safe laser angioplasty system. As seen in Figure 3–3, pulsed lasers appear to have an

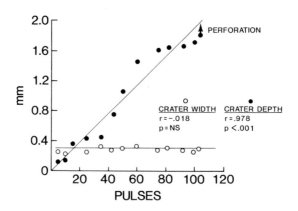

FIG 3–3.
Using ocular micrometry, a graph of the incision dimensions vs. the number of excimer pulses can be obtained. On the y axis is the depth or width in millimeters, and on the x axis is the number of pulses. This was done for 308-nm pulses at 30 mJ per pulse. There is a relatively linear relationship between depth and number of pulses. However, the width remains relatively constant. Precise control of depth without any change in width of a crater is possible and easily obtained, in contrast to the continuous-wave lasers, in which depth and width are only loosely correlated. (From Grundfest WS, Litvack F, Forrester JS, et al: Laser ablation of human atherosclerotic plaque without adjacent tissue injury. *J Am Coll Cardiol* 1985; 5:929–933. Reproduced by permission.)

inherent advantage over continuous-wave lasers, since the ablation by pulsed lasers removes a defined depth of tissue.[11]

Ablation by 7-nsec pulsed irradiation at 532 nm (the second harmonic of YAG laser) tends to produce variable results in atherosclerotic tissue. We observed many different outcomes of pulse 532-nm irradiation. Some tissues, particularly soft atheroma, appeared to undergo explosive ablation, as large particles were ejected from the tissue surface. Calcified tissue was relatively unaffected, and in some tissue specimens molten or liquid material filled the newly created hole, almost erasing all traces of irradiation. High-speed filming revealed tremendous scatter of the 532-nm radiation through the tissue. Similar processes were also observed at 1,040-nm irradiation. It should be pointed out that energies necessary to ablate calcified tissue at 532-nm energy pulses also destroy quartz plates. Therefore, it is indeed possible to ablate atheromatous tissue at 532 nm, but this is not a feasible solution for laser angioplasty since the energy density is in the gigawatt per square millimeter range and destroys all known fiberoptic schemes. In addition, such intense energies tend to produce severe blast injury within the tissues, causing complete loss of local tissue architecture (Plate 4). At shorter wavelengths, thresholds are lower and thermal and blast injury are minimized.

High-speed thermal analysis of the laser-tissue interaction has identified the temperatures at which tissue destruction occurs. Such thermal analysis is a relative measurement since it is not conducted under the conditions that occur in vivo. It does, however, allow us to predict the maximum temperatures that might occur in vivo. With this method of analysis, the thermal gradient and temperatures produced during the interaction of light with tissue can be studied and correlated with observed histologic findings. We see that irreversible protein denaturation (coagulation injury) occurs at temperatures in excess of 50 to 60° C. Above 100° C, blast injury becomes prominent. Above 125° C formation of carbon particles is seen. These processes, common to all continuous-wave lasers, are not seen when pulsed lasers are employed at optimal operating parameters.

During the analysis of pulsed 308-nm light with calcified atherosclerotic tissue, we observed a maximal temperature rise in vitro of 63.5° C. This was the maximum observed temperature in 395 specimens of eximer irradiated human cadaveric atherosclerotic aorta. In contrast, temperatures produced by argon, Nd:YAG, or continuous-wave ultraviolet sources exceeded 100° C in all cases (Fig 3–4). Figure 3–4 is a graph of the temperatures that occurred at 2 seconds during laser irradiation sufficient to produce a crater 1 mm deep. For continuous-wave Nd:YAG, argon, and ultraviolet lasers, temperatures always exceeded 125° C during the ablative process. In contrast, excimer ablation tem-

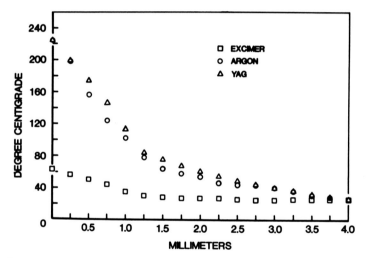

FIG 3–4.
Collating data, a graph of temperature vs. distance at 2 seconds for a given depth of ablation can be derived. On the x axis is distance from the crater center. The tissue has been set on the x and z axes extending into and out of the plane on the paper, and the laser is aimed on the y axis perpendicular to it. A crater 1 mm in diameter would have its edge at the 0.5 mm mark on this graph. For the neodymium (Nd)–YAG and the argon lasers, at the tissue edge the temperature is in excess of 100° C, and even at 1.5 mm the temperature is above 60° C. In contrast to the excimer laser, the temperature at 0.5 mm is less than 50° C, and within 1 mm the tissue temperature drops below 40° C. It is important to note that the tissue temperature barely exceeds 60° C, even in the center of the ablative excimer beam. This is important since 60° C is a temperature at which irreversible protein denaturation occurs. Thus, the excimer laser ablates tissue at temperatures much lower than those of the Nd:YAG or argon lasers.

peratures rarely exceeded 60° C. Laterally, only a small volume of tissue was heated above 50° C during excimer ablation. In contrast, a zone of tissue 1.5 to 2 mm in diameter was heated above 60° C during ablation with any of the continuous-wave sources.

Such widespread thermal heating accounts for the inability to control and precisely predict the events during direct continuous-wave radiation. Several schemes have been proposed to limit and confine thermal damage from continuous-wave sources. The most successful to date has been the use of the "hot-tip," which radially distributes the thermal energy over the vessel surface. Other devices are under investigation, including optical shields, sapphire tips, and defined ablation areas with multiple fibers, with the primary goal of preventing perforation due to uncontrolled thermal injury. To achieve meaningful experimental results, any analysis must be repeated, with the diversity of tissue samples ranging from smooth, mildly atherosclerotic atheroma to heavily calcified irregular disease. Failure to carry out analysis over a broad spectrum of biologic specimens will lead to a series of inappropriate conclusions.

As detailed by our angioscopic observations in coronary arteries, there is enormous variability even within a few centimeters of the arterial tree.[12] One section of the atheroma can be smooth and white and in the next centimeter the atheroma can be hard and calcified, followed by ulcerated, pigmented atheroma. Such heterogeneity makes it difficult to choose lasers based on a particular tissue characteristic. Attempts to achieve ablation through chromophore enhancement are limited by the tissue's variability or lack of chromophore uptake within many segments. Fifty percent to 60% of all coronary and 60% to 70% of all peripheral atheromas contain calcium. Very hard calcified lesions are not uncommon in either peripheral or coronary circulation. Thus, when choosing the appropriate laser for ablative processes, we must consider the tissue heterogeneity. None of the continuous-wave lasers, including carbon dioxide, Nd:YAG, argon ion, and continuous-wave ultraviolet, was effective in ablating calcified material. In contrast, the 308-nm excimer laser and the Nd:YAG 266-nm harmonic were capable of effective ablation of calcified material. Though 353 nm can ablate calcified material, this is somewhat more difficult and is accompanied by thermal injury in the surrounding tissue. At 532 nm, ablation of calcified material was almost impossible except at energy densities that exceeded 2 gigawatts/sq mm. This level of energy is clearly not feasible for fiberoptic transmission and is therefore impractical. Plate 5 demonstrates excimer ablation of a bovine femur. This was done through a fiberoptic waveguide in a saline medium. Note the preservation of the local tissue architecture on the smooth, clean cut that was possible using excimer ablation. It should be noted that if the energy level is subthreshold, thermal injury will occur.

The three-phase analytical method outlined above has allowed us to define the optimal wavelength for laser angioplasty by direct ablation. The optimal parameters for direct ablation appear to be in the pulsed ultraviolet wavelength. We have not yet tested the pulse and wavelength characteristics of the 2.9-μm lasers. Given the extremely short depth of penetration, one would predict that, through multiphoton processes, a precise ablative mechanism might occur at selected infrared wavelengths. However, fiber, lasers, and delivery systems have yet to be optimized for this wavelength.

ANIMAL MODELS FOR LASER ANGIOPLASTY

The next step in optimizing the laser-tissue interaction in regard to laser angioplasty is to study the healing response to laser irradiation. This can be performed in a variety of ways. There is as yet no good model for atherosclerosis in animals that allows observation of the healing response. We have, however, carried out studies in normal canine arteries. In addition, several investigators, including Abela et al.[13] and Sanborn et al.,[14] have studied the effects of various continuous wavelengths on normal canine arteries as well as atherosclerotic arteries in rabbits. Each of these models has its advantages and disadvantages. The studies in normal arteries allow one to predict the human response for relatively normal human vasculature and look for thrombus formation and intimal proliferation resulting from endothelial cell injury. In addition, such normal models can be used to study the potential for aneurysm formation. However, these models are only relative predictors of the healing response that such lasers will have in man.

Experiments in atherosclerotic rabbits allow investigators to evaluate the ability of a particular laser to ablate soft, smooth, toothpastelike atheroma and to test for the potential of perforation, since rabbit arteries are very thin. However, rabbit atherosclerosis is a foam-cell disease. It is not directly comparable to the human atherosclerotic process. Several investigators have implanted excised human coronary arteries into dogs; however, the intense fibrotic reaction due to the foreign body makes study of healing responses difficult to interpret.[13] We have developed a different model that appears to simulate fibrotic human atherosclerosis.[15] This model permits one to assess the flexibility and ability of systems to recanalize vessels similar to coronary arteries. This model is too new, though, to permit the study of the laser-tissue interaction since it takes approximately 4 to 6 months for the atherosclerotic process to develop. Once the characteristics of this model have been quantified, it may allow for a better understanding of the healing processes that occur in the presence of smooth muscle cell proliferation.

COMPARISON OF IN VIVO THERMAL AND HISTOLOGIC EFFECTS OF ARGON AND EXCIMER

Previous research has demonstrated that 308-nm excimer laser light ablates vascular tissue with great precision and minimal thermal effect. However, lack of a fiberoptic delivery system has limited study of in vivo effect of excimer lasers.

To define acute and chronic histologic differences produced by excimer and argon ablation delivered by fiberoptics in living animals, and to correlate these histologic effects with thermal gradients produced by ablation in vascular tissue, we studied laser effects in vivo.[16, 17] In 25 anesthetized dogs, we employed a standardized method of aortic exposure through a midline incision. Through the midline incision, the abdominal aorta was controlled and the posterior intima exposed by a longitudinal aortotomy. Irradiation of a 125-sq mm area within a template was performed. Eight aortas were irradiated with argon laser and 13 aortas were irradiated with an excimer laser. In four control dogs the aorta was opened, exposed, and repaired but not irradiated. Aortic repair was performed with 6-0 polypropylene (Prolene). A 308-nm excimer laser was delivered through a 600-μm core fiberoptic waveguide in contact with the tissue. Argon laser energy was transmitted by a 400-μm core fiber held 5 ± 2 mm from the intimal surface. Excimer spot size was 0.6 mm in diameter. Argon spot size was 0.6 to 0.7 mm in diameter. Energy density was 25 to 35 mJ/sq mm per pulse at 20 Hz for the excimer laser, or 0.5 to 0.7 J/sq mm/second. Argon energy was delivered at 5.1 to 15.5 J/sq mm/second. Irradiation was continued until the intimal surface in the template was ablated.

Three methods of analysis were used. First was immediate gross appearance as photographed, with the surface characterized as smooth, irregular, or carbonized. Second, during irradiation thermal gradients were recorded with a thermal camera (AGA 782). Third, serial histology was obtained from acute response to 4-week healing.

Acute continuous-wave irradiated aorta showed carbonization and thermal destruction of adjacent tissue. Excimer-irradiated specimens showed no gross evidence of thermal injury. Temperature measurement showed argon ablation occurring above 115° C (Plate 6). In contrast, excimer ablative temperatures did not exceed 48° C (Plate 7). At three days, argon-irradiated aortas all revealed mural thrombus with an inflammatory infiltrate visible on histologic examination. Excimer-irradiated aortas showed minimal thrombus, no inflammatory response, and new islands of endothelial cells.

The most striking difference occurred at 4 weeks. Argon-irradiated aortas were surrounded by dense inflammatory response and showed evidence of minimal hyperplasia, with disorganization of subendothelial components. Excimer-irradiated aortas were grossly similar to controls, with a normally reconstituted endothelium and an intact internal elastic lamina on histologic examination.

As the above study was performed in canine arteries, its relevance to atherosclerotic arteries is unclear. The available data suggest that the significant trauma to the vessel wall leads to platelet aggregation and a subsequent proliferative response. The magnitude of the "healing response" is in part due to the magnitude of injury. Thus, it seems likely that lasers that cut with minimal adjacent tissue damage will produce a surface less likely to cause restenosis and thrombosis. This remains to be tested in the clinical setting.

REFERENCES

1. Gorisch W, Boargen KP: Heat induced contraction of blood vessels. *Lasers Surg Med* 1982; 2:1–13.
2. Anderson RR, Parrish JA: Selective photothermolysis: Precise microsurgery by selective absorption of pulsed radiation. *Science* 1983; 220:524–527.
3. Hu C, Barnes FS: The thermal-chemical damage in biological material under laser irradiation. *IEEE Trans Biomed Eng* 1970; 17:220–231.
4. Srinivasan R: Ablation of polymers and biological tissues by ultraviolet lasers. *Science* 1986; 234:559–565.
5. Spears JR, Serur J, Shropstire D, et al: Fluorescence of experimental atheromatous plaques with hematoporphyrin derivative. *J Clin Invest* 1983; 71:395–399.
6. Litvack F, Grundfest WS, Forrester JS, et al: Effects of hematoporphyrin derivative and photodynamic therapy on arteriosclerotic rabbits. *Am J Cardiol* 1985; 56:667–671.
7. Abela GS, Barbieri E, Roxey T, et al: Laser enhanced plaque atherolysis with tetracycline, abstracted. *Circulation* 1986; 72(suppl 2):7.
8. Prince MR, Deutsch TF, Mathews-Roth MM, et al: Preferential light absorption in atheromas in vitro: Implications for laser angioplasty. *J Clin Invest* 1986; 78:295–302.
9. Cothren RM, Hayes GB, Cramer JR, et al: A multifiber catheter with an optical shield for laser angiosurgery. *Lasers Life Sci* 1987; 1:1–12.
10. Sartori MP, Bossaller C, Weilbacher D, et al: Detection of atherosclerotic plaques and characterization of arterial wall structure by laser induced fluorescence, abstracted. *Circulation* 1986; 74(suppl 2):7.
11. Grundfest WS, Litvack F, Forrester JS, et al: Laser ablation of human atherosclerotic plaque without adjacent tissue injury. *J Am Coll Cardiol* 1985; 5:929–933.
12. Forrester JS, Litvack F, Grundfest W, et al: A perspective of coronary disease seen through the arteries of living man. *Circulation* 1987; 75:505–513.
13. Abela GS, Normann SJ, Cohen DM, et al: Laser recanalization of occluded atherosclerotic arteries in vivo and in vitro. *Circulation* 1985; 71:403–411.
14. Sanborn TA, Faxon DP, Haudenschild C, et al: Experimental angioplasty—Circumferential distributions of laser thermal energy with a laser probe. *J Am Coll Cardiol* 1985; 5:934.
15. Doyle L, Litvack F, Grundfest W, et al: An in vivo model for testing laser angioplasty systems, abstracted. *Circulation* 1986; 74(suppl 2):361.
16. Grundfest WS, Litvack F, Doyle L, et al: Comparison of in vitro and in vivo thermal effects of argon and excimer lasers for laser angioplasty, abstracted. *Circulation* 1986; 74(suppl 2):204.
17. Litvack F, Doyle L, Grundfest W, et al: In vivo excimer laser ablation: Acute and chronic effects of canine aorta, abstracted. *Circulation* 1986; 74(suppl 2):360.

4

Laser Angioplasty Delivery Systems: Design Considerations

Martin B. Leon, M.D.
Paul D. Smith, Ph.D.
Robert F. Bonner, Ph.D.

Since the advent and widespread use of percutaneous transluminal balloon angioplasty in the late 1970s and 1980s,[1] investigators and clinicians have pondered the next generation of catheter-based devices that would expand our ability to remodel obstructed coronary and peripheral arteries. Certainly the most popular, and probably the most promising, of these new technologies employs concentrated light energy from lasers via small, flexible optical fibers to a distant intravascular target site to vaporize or ablate atherosclerotic lesions. Laser angioplasty represents a natural progression stemming from (1) the already established role of lasers as microsurgical ablative instruments in ophthalmology, dermatology, and general surgery; (2) the realization that definitive arterial recanalization may frequently require tissue debulking or removal; and (3) the development of current interventional balloon techniques. The success of laser angioplasty as a therapeutic modality in the future will depend on a convincing demonstration that, compared with balloon angioplasty techniques, safe laser plaque ablation can improve the risk profile, reduce the frequency of restenosis, and expand the range of patient candidates.

The purpose of this chapter is to discuss the physical principles and practical considerations that underlie the fabrication of multifunctional laser catheter delivery systems for laser angioplasty. It bears emphasizing that clinical

44

trials using prototype laser angioplasty devices have only recently been initiated; therefore, the contents of this chapter are based largely on in vitro data and preclinical animal investigations.

AN INTEGRATED APPROACH

Enthusiasm for the potential benefits of laser angioplasty must be viewed in the sobering context of possible disturbing complications, including acute thrombus formation, particulate embolization, and most importantly, inadvertent arterial wall perforation. Early animal experiments[2-4] and preliminary clinical trials in patients with peripheral and coronary artery disease[5-7] have resulted in an unacceptable frequency of vessel wall perforation. Given the high-risk nature of these procedures, it seems proper to demand that future laser angioplasty systems (1) be capable of ablating variable-composition atheroma (fatty, fibrous, and calcified lesions); (2) induce tissue vaporization with high efficiency such that radial thermal transfer to surrounding normal tissue is limited; (3) create an ablated surface that favors rapid healing and reendothelialization with minimal thrombogenicity; (4) remove tissue without generation of particulate debris sufficient in size to cause cytotoxic or ischemic sequelae; (5) provide a means of plaque recognition and feedback control to improve target site specificity; (6) transmit the energy through small, flexible, durable optical fibers that have a low risk of being damaged by energy densities required to ablate plaque; (7) incorporate the optical fibers and feedback control within a catheter-based delivery system of requisite size and steerability to safely negotiate the small, tortuous conduits of the distal coronary and peripheral arterial circulations. Perhaps the technologies necessary to produce this theoretical catheter delivery system are not yet fully developed, but useful lessons can be derived from a critical examination of current and proposed laser angioplasty prototype devices.

Most investigators agree that an ideal delivery system will require an integrated approach involving three major components: the laser-fiberoptic, a multifunctional catheter, and a guidance-control unit (Fig 4–1). Although the entire

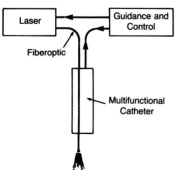

FIG 4–1.
An integrated system for laser angioplasty including a laser-fiberoptic, a multifunctional catheter, and a guidance and control unit, which both receives information from the target site and interacts with the laser source.

system may be viewed as modular, the components are interdependent as each has impact on design features of the others. Importantly, minimum standards must be met by each of the major components. For example, if the effects of a given laser-fiberoptic combination result in thrombogenic surfaces and transmural thermal or acoustic damage to the vessel wall, then the most elaborate guidance-control system will be unable to provide the clinical operator with an efficacious tool.

An important design consideration for laser angioplasty delivery systems is an understanding of the specific clinical situations and proposed tasks required of the instrument. Clearly, design execution must be far more meticulous if the goal is definitive vessel recanalization as a procedure standing alone (i.e., laser endarterectomy) vs. laser-assisted balloon angioplasty, wherein laser ablation of plaque reestablishes a small primary channel that is subsequently enlarged by balloon dilation. Similarly, intraoperative laser angioplasty may always be safer than the percutaneous route, and the hazards associated with working in the coronary circulation will always impose special constraints compared with larger and less tortuous peripheral arteries. The ultimate goal is to perform definitive percutaneous laser coronary angioplasty. Unfortunately, present technology requires considerable additional refinement before this objective can be achieved at an acceptable risk to patients.

LASER-FIBEROPTIC SELECTION

The choice of laser wavelength has evoked widespread controversy, and there is no general agreement among investigators that a single laser-fiberoptic combination is clearly superior. However, an understanding of fundamental principles of laser tissue vaporization and fiberoptic transmission combined with a critical examination of available in vitro data helps to clarify advantages and limitations of currently proposed laser-fiberoptic systems.

Concepts of Laser Tissue Vaporization

Laser light incident on a target tissue is usually absorbed by molecules (chromophores) and converted into thermal energy. The local deposition of thermal energy can cause tissue coagulation (denaturation of structural proteins), melting of lipid or other tissue components (solid or gel to liquid phase transitions), or explosive vaporization if the heat of vaporization for tissue is rapidly realized (roughly 2 J/cu mm). For any laser source, the rapidity and degree of tissue heating depends on competing processes, including thermal diffusion and convection, which results in heat loss to the surrounding environment. Efficient tissue ablation occurs when most of the laser energy is deposited and retained in the zone of tissue subsequently vaporized. Conversely, inefficient tissue ablation occurs when there are significant heat losses, either into surrounding, nonablated tissue due to thermal diffusion or into the fluid operating medium (i.e., blood or crystalloid perfusate) due to convection. Thermal diffusion depends on the rate at which molecules transfer energy to neighboring molecules and is determined by the tissue absorption characteristics of light at a given wavelength. In a fluid medium, heat loss due to convection is often much greater than heat loss from thermal diffusion; hence, most laser angioplasty systems are designed to maintain fiber-tissue contact, thereby reducing exposure to fluid interfaces and minimizing convective loss. Accordingly, in a contact mode of operation, thermal diffusion is usually the principal cause of reduced lasing efficiency and is responsible for thermal tissue injury in border zones surrounding sites of laser vaporization.

Since thermal diffusion is a physical process that can be quantitated, one can predict and model tissue heating and vaporization patterns for different laser wavelengths and lasing parameters (i.e., power, spot size, and pulse duration). Although such models are merely theoretical constructs that may not be entirely valid under in vivo situations, they serve as helpful guidelines to compare important properties of different lasers. Assuming that the light energy is absorbed in tissue as a linear process, energy deposition is determined by the absorption coefficient, α, for each wavelength (Fig 4–2). Based on previous carbon dioxide (CO_2) laser ophthalmology experiments,[8] for efficient tissue vaporization (>50% of the total energy vaporizes a zone to a depth of $1/\alpha$), the surface pulse energy density should be roughly three.times the ablative threshold, or $6,000/\alpha$ J/sq cm, for a pulse duration of $900/\alpha^2$ seconds or less. From these formulae, approximate values can be generated for ablation depth per pulse, pulse duration, energy density (or fluence), and thermal damage for efficient vaporization as a function of wavelength. These data allow comparisons between different lasers and help to specify the requirements of transmitting optical fibers. As a practical consideration, strong tissue absorption of light (i.e., higher absorption coefficients) favors efficient thermal ablation at a lower energy density and results in a smaller zone of thermal tissue injury

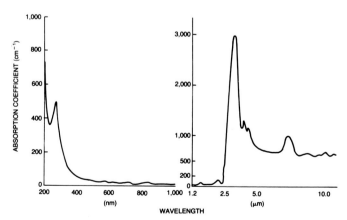

FIG 4–2.
The absorption spectra of human necropsy atherosclerotic plaque.

while requiring a shorter pulse duration. These relationships are corroborated by histologic data that indicate thermal ablation can be performed more efficiently with minimal thermal damage to surrounding tissue zones at laser wavelengths with a higher tissue absorption coefficient.[9, 10]

Many conditions may modify these approximations for thermal ablation by lasers: (1) convective losses may assume greater importance than thermal diffusion, particularly in a wet field for longer pulse durations or repetitive pulses,[8] and/or when the fiber and target tissue are not in direct contact; (2) for hard tissues, such as calcified plaque, thermal ablation may be a less efficient or even an ineffective means of tissue removal (i.e., if the force generated by vaporization of tissue water cannot disrupt calcified structures); (3) absorption characteristics of the tissue may change during a pulse or pulse sequence, thereby changing ablation efficiency; (4) rapid fiber advancement during tissue ablation may reduce thermal injury if tissue ablation proceeds as quickly as thermal diffusion (especially true for continuous argon lasers); and (5) ablative efficiency may be increased by lasers that cause tissue ablation by nonthermal mechanisms. This last point requires further elaboration. Excimer lasers may initiate tissue ablation by direct breaking of chemical bonds by high-energy photons (so-called photochemical effects).[11] Alternatively, several lasers capable of producing high peak powers at the tissue surface during short pulses ($\leq 10^{-6}$ seconds) may cause nonlinear absorption of light energy, resulting in plasma formation and/or acoustic shock wave effects, which can improve ablative efficiency.[12, 13]

Optical Fibers

Optical fibers can transmit light with very low losses over great distances and are a critical design component in all laser angioplasty delivery systems. In fact, without small, flexible, durable, low-loss fibers, the concept of catheter-based percutaneous intravascular laser ablation of atheromatous lesions at distant sites in the coronary tree or peripheral circulation would be inconceivable. Although a rigid waveguide (either hand-held or coupled to an articulated arm) may be used as a transmission vehicle for laser light over short distances, clinical applications are restricted to intraoperative settings where the target lesions are directly visualized or accessible to manual palpation.

Physics of Fiber Transmission

Optical fibers for laser light transmission consist of a central core material that is essentially transparent at the operating wavelength, an overcoating or cladding, and an outer coating, usually referred to as a jacket or sheath. The cladding has a refractive index less than but close to the refractive index of the core fiber. Cladding provides a means to isolate the core from the environment, which enables handling the fiber without causing surface changes at the core interface. Cladding also helps to minimize transmission losses associated with fiber defects or with bending of the fiber and assists the designer in

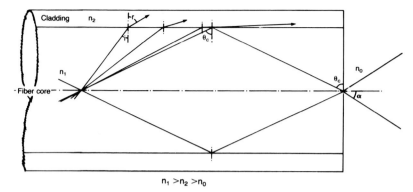

FIG 4–3.
Snell's law: $n_1\sin(i) = n_2\sin(r)$, where n is the refractive index of the medium and i and r are the angles of incidence and refraction. The critical angle, Θ_c, is the smallest angle of incidence at which total internal reflection occurs. The numerical aperture is $n_o\sin(\alpha)$ and is determined by Θ_c.

controlling the propagation characteristics of the fiber. The jacket serves no purpose in light transmission but is essential to the mechanical integrity of the fiber.

Two principles that are important in understanding light transmission through fibers are total internal reflection and numerical aperture. Snell's law of refraction, which governs the relationship of light propagation at media interfaces, states that $n_1\sin(i) = n_2\sin(r)$, where i and r are the angles of incidence and refraction and n is the refractive index of the medium (Fig 4–3). As the angle of incidence is increased, an angle known as the critical angle (θ_c) is reached where the refracted ray is tangential to the surface ($r = 90°$). For greater angles of incidence, total internal reflection occurs and all light is reflected at the core-cladding interface back into the central core along the entire length of the fiber. It is apparent that by changing the refractive indexes of the cladding and core material, the critical angle at which total internal reflection occurs can be adjusted, thus determining the smallest angle of incidence that can propagate down the fiber. The total internal reflection process is virtually loss-free, and attenuation through the fiber for the short distances involved in medical applications depends on light absorption by the fiber material at the wavelength of propagation.

The numerical aperture of the fiber is also dictated by the refractive indexes of the core and cladding and determines both the cone of light accepted by the input surface of the fiber and the cone of light emerging from the output surface. The numerical aperture of the fiber is $n_o\sin(\alpha)$, where α is the half angle of the acceptance or emergence cone (see Fig 4–3). The numerical aperture is critical for coupling light into the fiber; thus, if a laser beam is focused coaxially onto the fiber core (spot size less than core diameter) with a numerical aperture less than the numerical aperture of the fiber, the light will be totally internally reflected and the only losses will be associated with absorption within the core and reflection at the end surfaces. Moreover, by establishing the beam divergence patterns from the output surface, numerical aperture of the fiber defines the power or energy density at the tissue a given distance from the fiber tip.

As the power in a laser pulse is progressively increased, invariably a point will be reached at which the optical fiber will be damaged. Beyond this fiber damage threshold, laser light transmission diminishes suddenly owing to high local losses at the point of breakdown within the fiber. Fiber breakdown falls into two general categories: (1) material properties of the fiber core determining local absorption at different wavelengths (especially important when operating in the ultraviolet or infrared); and (2) manufacturing defects of the fiber, such as microscopic surface scratches along the fiber shaft or cleavage defects at the input or output surfaces. Also, abrupt bends in small fibers, as might be required in the coronary circulation, can alter internal reflection patterns, leading to local losses, heating, and ultimately breakdown of the fiber. Finally, lasers capable of generating high peak power densities (approaching 1 gigawatt/sq cm) can induce fiber damage by nonlinear mechanisms associated with plasma formation at the input or output surface.

Properties of Optical Fibers

An optical fiber should be chosen for a laser source on the basis of its transparency at the operating wavelength, its numerical aperture, the degree of cladding losses, and its resistance to damage at high powers (Table 4–1). In addition, size, flexibility, durability, and biocompatibility are important variables in fiber selection. The mechanical properties of a fiber depend on the material and the fiber diameter. For a given material; (1) the force required to bend the fiber increases as the fourth power of the fiber diameter (stiffness αd^4); (2) the minimal radius of curvature of a fiber before breaking varies as the fiber diameter (flexibility $\alpha 1/d$); and (3) the power-transmitting capacity of the fiber increases with the square of the fiber diameter. However, other factors can partially override the purely physical characteristics of the fiber ma-

TABLE 4–1.
Properties of 0.2-mm-Diameter Optical Fibers

MATERIAL	WAVELENGTH, μM	FLEXIBILITY, CM BEND RADIUS	DAMAGE, W IN CW MODE*	OTHER†
Silica	0.3–2.1	0.3	20	1, 2, 3, 4
Borosilicate	0.38–1.5	0.3	10	1, 2, 3, 4
Zirconium fluoride	0.34–5.0	1.0	20	2, 3(?), 4, 5
Chalcogenide	1.0–5.0, 2.0–11.0	1.0	10	3(?), 4, 5
Silver halide	0.5–11.0	High loss‡	20	5, 6

*CW indicates continuous wave.
†1 indicates commercial; 2, durable; 3, biocompatible; 4, glass (drawn); 5, developmental; 6, extruded.
‡Not clad so that high local loss results from abrupt bends.

terial. For instance, the jacket material can both enhance the tensile strength of the fiber and act as a strain relief in sharp bends. Nevertheless, the above fiber property relationships indicate that as stiffness decreases and flexibility increases with decreasing fiber diameter, at the same time the power-transmitting capacity of the fiber is correspondingly reduced. As a practical consideration, for almost all materials currently available, fiber stiffness precludes the use of single fibers with core diameters greater than 0.4 mm. Clearly, for laser angioplasty, a compromise in fiber selection between size, flexibility, stiffness, and transmitting capacity must be made to provide the necessary maneuverability and torque control of the catheter delivery system while maintaining sufficient power output to ablate variable-composition atheroma.

Comparison of Laser-Fiberoptic Systems

The earliest argon laser-fiberoptic systems used for crude angioplasty experiments[14, 15] and for preliminary clinical trials[5–7] were not selected on the basis of a critical analysis of laser-tissue interactions, but rather were chosen owing to the convenience of transmitting argon laser wavelengths through low-loss commercial glass fibers. An understanding of the advantages and limitations of argon laser systems has stimulated extensive investigation seeking to optimize ablation efficiency of atheroma by choosing different laser sources.

A critical determinant of all laser-fiberoptic combinations is an appreciation of the operating range of the system (Fig 4–4). The operating range for a

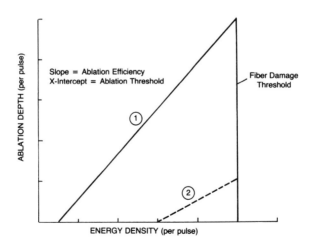

FIG 4–4.
By plotting ablation depth vs. pulse energy density, the operating range for a laser-fiberoptic system can be defined as the pulse energy densities between the fiber damage threshold and the ablation threshold for soft tissue (x intercept). Ablation efficiency of the system is represented as the slope of the relationship. System 1 has a favorable operating range and a high ablation efficiency, whereas system 2 has a narrow operating range and a low ablation efficiency.

given laser and fiberoptic is defined as the pulse energy densities between the threshold required for soft-tissue ablation and the threshold at which fiber damage occurs. By plotting ablation depth vs. pulse energy density, the ablation efficiency of a system can also be characterized, assuming linear mechanisms of tissue ablation (see Fig 4–4). Since efficient thermal ablation requires an energy density approximately three times the ablative threshold for soft tissue, and calcified atheroma increases the ablative threshold while reducing ablation efficiency, a favorable laser-fiberoptic combination for clinical biomedical applications should have a maximal operating range approximately ten times the ablative threshold.

Comparisons of both conventional and developmental laser-fiberoptic systems are summarized in Table 4–2. If one could design the "ideal" laser and fiberoptic for ablative angioplasty, the following criteria would be fulfilled: (1) either selective plaque ablation or superficial energy absorption resulting in efficient thermal vaporization with minimal radial thermal diffusion; (2) capable by thermal or nonthermal mechanisms of ablating calcified atheroma; (3) a wide energy density operating range for the laser wavelength and fiberoptic; and (4) commercially available low-loss fiberoptics with acceptable size, flexibility, and durability properties. At present, none of the proposed systems fulfills all of these criteria.

Excimer

Operating in the ultraviolet, in the nanosecond (nsec) pulse range, commercial fused silica fibers can transmit 308-nm excimer laser pulses to elicit precise microablative effects without thermal tissue injury in fatty, fibrous, and calcified atheroma. The mechanisms of tissue ablation are probably a combi-

TABLE 4–2.
Proposed Laser-Fiberoptic Systems*

LASER	WAVELENGTH, NM	PULSE DURATION	PRINCIPAL FIBER	PLAQUE ABLATION		OPERATING RANGE	OTHER†
				EFFICIENCY	CALCIFIED		
Excimer	248			H	Y	?	3, 4
	308	2–200 nsec	Silica	H	Y	L	3, 4 (?)
	351			M-H	Y (?)	L	4
Argon	488, 512	40 msec–CW	Silica	L-M	N	M-H	1
Dye laser	450–800	1–2 μsec	Silica	M	?	M	1, 4
Nd:YAG	1,064	10^{-9}–10^{-12} sec	None	H	N (?)	0	4
		CW	Silica	L	N	M-H	1
Ho:YLF	2,060	100 μsec	Silica	M	?	M-H (?)	2
Er:YAG	2,940	100 μsec	ZrF$_4$	H	Y	H	2, 5
CO$_2$	10,600	1 μsec	Halide (?)	H	Y (?)	?	2, 4, 5
		10 msec	Halide	M-H	N	L	2, 5
		CW	Halide	L	N	L	1, 2, 5

*H indicates high; Y, yes; L, low; M, medium; CW, continuous wave; N, no; Nd, neodymium; Ho, holmium; Er, erbium.
†1 indicates extensive thermal damage; 2, strong water absorption; 3, possible mutagenicity; 4, nonthermal ablative mechanisms; 5, developmental fibers.

nation of photothermal and poorly understood photochemical effects. Since light is absorbed by protein and nucleic acid chromophores (and not water), another advantage may be retained ablation efficiency in crystalloid media allowing the possibility of tissue ablation without fiber-target contact. Theoretical disadvantages include mutagenicity concerns at ultraviolet wavelengths, halogen gas hazards in a clinical environment, and a narrow energy density operating range. New developments in pulse-stretched excimer lasers (200-nsec to 1-μsec pulses) will reduce peak power densities, thus widening the operating range by increasing the threshold for fiber damage.

Argon

Operating in the visible, usually in the continuous or mechanically chopped mode, argon lasers transmitted via silica fibers have a favorable operating range and can be transmitted through a crystalloid medium, but ablation efficiency is low, with marked surrounding thermal damage in soft tissues. These systems cannot ablate calcified lesions. Thermal diffusion can be minimized by increased laser power density, shortened exposure times (to <1 second), and rapid forward advancement of the fiber during tissue ablation. However, the rapid ablation velocities needed to reduce thermal diffusion also diminish operator control, which predisposes to transmural perforation.

Dye Lasers

Tunable dye lasers (450 to 800 nm) operating in a short pulse mode are moderately efficient for soft-tissue ablation owing to relatively poor absorption of visible light by vascular tissue. High peak powers may increase fiber damage thresholds, thereby narrowing the operating range. On the other hand, the short, high-power pulses may improve ablative efficiency by nonlinear mechanisms and may disrupt calcified material by plasma formation and shock-wave generation. Data are preliminary, but shock waves from high-power pulses may also be disadvantageous; large tissue fragments and extensive arterial wall damage have been observed.

Neodymium:YAG

Continuous neodymium:yttrium-aluminum-garnet (Nd:YAG) lasers are poorly suited for ablative angioplasty. Despite a wide operating range, ablative efficiency is extremely low and calcified lesions are unaffected. Intense thermal tissue changes are more useful for nonablative applications, such as laser tissue welding for microvascular anastomoses. Short-pulse Nd:YAG lasers may ablate soft tissue efficiently by nonlinear mechanisms, but fiber transmission is not practical.

Holmium–YLF

Although still developmental, these lasers take advantage of a weak water absorption peak and may be useful in the future. Operating in the near-infrared spectrum, absorption coefficients are three times greater than with visible wavelengths, resulting in slightly improved ablation efficiency. Fiber transmission through commercial silica is possible, and the operating range may be favorable. Disadvantages include uncertainty concerning calcified plaque removal and the requirement of fiber-target contact in a fluid operating medium.

Erbium (Er)–YAG

In this instance, both the laser and especially the fibers are developmental. Nevertheless, very strong water absorption at 2.9 μm provides excellent ablative efficiency with minimal thermal damage to the artery wall. Ablation of calcified material has been demonstrated, and if preliminary data using zirconium fluoride fibers are reproducible, the operating range is most favorable. Theoretically, commercial-grade fibers can be fabricated to the requisite design specifications; however, flexibility is a problem. The Er:YAG laser system may have an important role in clinical ablative angioplasty. The major apparent disadvantage is water-based absorption, which necessitates fiber-target contact for intravascular ablation.

CO_2

Carbon dioxide lasers also utilize water absorption for ablation and may be operated in a variety of pulse modes. Importantly, fiber transmission is problematic; developmental halide and chalcogenide fibers are thus far neither small enough nor flexible enough to be incorporated within catheter delivery systems. Continuous CO_2 lasers can cause thermal tissue injury and cannot ablate calcified lesions. Short-pulse CO_2 lasers (especially the microsecond transversely excited laser) elicit highly efficient ablative effects and can remove calcified plaques. Again, water-based absorption requires direct fiber-target contact to achieve tissue ablation.

MULTIFUNCTIONAL CATHETER DESIGNS

The clinical utility of new catheters for laser angioplasty will depend on imaginative design concepts providing for the safe delivery of laser energy via optical fibers to intravascular target sites without greatly altering the catheter properties that have been applied successfully in balloon angioplasty. One should take advantage of the many design and fabrication lessons learned to achieve a distal catheter position in the coronary and systemic circulations during more than a decade of experience with balloon angioplasty.

In the peripheral arterial circulation, vessels are larger and straighter and have a normally higher ratio of media to intima thickness compared with the coronary arteries, which improves tensile strength of the vessel wall. These anatomic characteristics contribute to a reduced likelihood of transmural perforation during laser angioplasty. Moreover, the immediate and long-term consequences of inadvertent perforation can usually be managed with minimal patient risk, except in the situation of a major iliac artery perforation. Catheters should be composed of nonthrombogenic materials; shaft size will vary (from 4 to 9 F) depending on surrounding vessel lumen caliber and intended application (either stand-alone procedure or laser-assisted balloon angioplasty); and column rigidity of the catheter should be sufficient to provide adequate support or "backup" both to maintain torque control and to advance the catheter system through long segments of total occlusions. Unless operating in the more distal posterior tibial circulation, tip flexibility, low profile designs, and steerability issues are of less importance.

In contrast, laser angioplasty in the smaller, more tortuous epicardial coronary arteries presents far greater engineering and fabrication challenges. Catheters should also be composed of nonthrombogenic materials; shaft outer diameter cannot exceed 1.5 mm (between 4 and 5 F); and column rigidity must still be sufficient to engage and cross severely stenotic or totally occluded lesions. Since positioning the catheter at a distal site may require navigating around one or more sharp vessel bends or branch points, flexibility, stiffness, steerability, and catheter tip configuration assume critical importance. Therefore, an over-the-wire design, as is used in current balloon angioplasty systems, would be a helpful adjunct to laser angioplasty catheters. Teflon-coated guidewires (0.014 to 0.018 in. outside diameter [OD]) are atraumatic, can be preformed to improve steerability, and ensure coaxial positioning of the catheter, which reduces the risks of perforation. Similarly, a catheter for the coronary arteries must have a bend radius at the tip of 5 mm or less and should have distal lumen for dye injections and measurement of translesional pressure gradients. The distal catheter tip may require tapering for laser-assisted balloon angioplasty or may retain the shaft diameter if a maximal ablative surface is preferable during laser stand-alone procedures. Clearly, to incorporate all of these design features in a catheter that also must accommodate optical fibers for laser light transmission as well as a guidance and control unit becomes an engineering tour de force.

Perhaps the simplest laser catheter designs for use in both peripheral and coronary arteries incorporate a fixed or movable central optical fiber within a catheter.[16] A more useful system would include a surrounding balloon catheter for coaxial positioning and for laser-assisted balloon angioplasty.[17] This over-the-fiber design may have limited clinical applications owing to the large fiber size required (0.5 to 1.0 mm OD) to advance the balloon catheter through the primary channel, which markedly reduces catheter tip flexibility and predisposes to mechanical vessel wall perforation.[5–7, 18] The development of fiber bundles (large numbers of small fibers closely packed in a common sheath) might improve catheter flexibility and diminish these risks. However, it becomes more complicated to couple laser energy into a fiber bundle, and individual fiber damage may trigger catastrophic system failure.

An important consideration in laser catheter fabrication is the problem of creating a channel that is considerably larger than the cross-sectional area of the catheter tip. This becomes less critical in laser-assisted balloon angioplasty, wherein a channel only large enough to introduce a balloon catheter for subsequent dilation is required. However, when laser angioplasty is a stand-alone procedure in peripheral or coronary arteries, definitive recanalization will necessitate an expanded ablative surface. Clinical investigators and catheter design engineers have proposed several possible solutions to this problem. If the laser catheter is withdrawn a small distance from the target lesion, the cone of light emerging from the fiber will diverge, resulting in a larger spot size than the fiber itself. The requirements of a noncontact laser catheter include the following: (1) it must have a sufficiently high fiber numerical aperture (i.e., a numerical aperture of 0.2 and a catheter-tissue separation of 5 mm are required to double the ablative diameter of a 1.5-mm catheter); (2) the laser wavelength must be transparent for the operating medium; and (3) the system operating range must be large enough to maintain efficient tissue ablation (a twofold increase in ablative diameter results in a fourfold decrease in energy density at the target). These requirements become almost insoluble limitations when one considers that blood absorbs and scatters all laser wavelengths. Although excimer wavelengths (308 and 351 nm) are transparent to crystalloid solutions, the present operating range is too narrow to permit more than a twofold or threefold drop in target energy density with beam expansion before fiber breakdown occurs. Furthermore, distance between the fiber tip and the target site is difficult to control, resulting in variable tissue dosimetry and inconsistent ablative effects. Therefore, most new laser catheter designs utilize fiber-target contact to minimize the effects of the intervening operating medium and to deliver reproducible tissue dosimetry for more predictable atheroma ablation. Another technique to enlarge the ablative surface consists of repetitive overlapping laser exposures in close proximity, which can be accomplished by rotating the catheter around either a central or an eccentric guide wire.

Recently, considerable attention has been directed toward modifications in catheter tip configurations. These developments have grown from the observation that heated metallic-tip catheters can effectively recanalize obstructed human atherosclerotic lesions in peripheral arteries with an unexpectedly low risk of vessel wall perforation.[19–21] Many laser catheter designs use a small (≤3 mm) optical shield (or window), which is bonded to the catheter shaft, is composed of transmitting optical materials (usually quartz or sapphire), and can be fabricated in a variety of geometric forms (hemisphere, cylinder, or cone). A rounded optical shield presents a less traumatic surface to the intima, which reduces the likelihood of mechanical perforation from bare fibers. The shield material may also be more durable than the core fiber and present no chemical toxicity. Other advantages include a target spot size larger than the fiber diameter, since the fiber is now further from the target, and a variety of laser beam profiles. Thus, smaller, more flexible fibers may be employed to ablate larger tissue surfaces. It should be noted that the use of optical shields in laser catheters is not without problems and demands substantial fabrication expertise; reflection from the input surface of the shield, bonding to the catheter shaft, reduced catheter tip flexibility (especially with longer shields), and

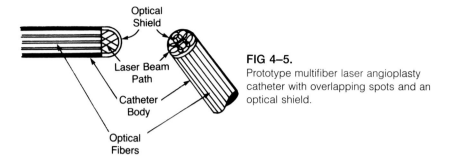

FIG 4–5.
Prototype multifiber laser angioplasty catheter with overlapping spots and an optical shield.

difficulties with central over-the-wire designs must all be accounted for during catheter construction.

Finally, several investigators have proposed multifiber catheters as a means to increase catheter shaft and/or tip flexibility while providing a large ablative surface.[22] Catheters have already been constructed with 4 to 19 small optical fibers (80 to 150 μm OD) in a concentric dense-pack or separated array, such that nearest neighbor fibers create overlapping spots, resulting in a honeycombing appearance of the ablated surface (Fig 4–5). Depending on the complexity of the system, each fiber (or group of fibers) may be fired individually and serially, thereby illuminating only a small portion of the composite spot at any given time. Sequential firing of individual fibers with proper timing between repetitive pulses may reduce thermal injury from lasers by allowing time for thermal relaxation between successive laser exposures. Multifiber laser catheter designs are largely determined by the choice of laser and transmitting optical fiber. For instance, since excimer lasers produce superficial tissue ablation without important thermal injury, sequential firing of fibers becomes unnecessary. However, the narrow operating range of excimer lasers limits the possibility of significant beam expansion, thus requiring a closely packed array of fibers positioned near the catheter tip. Conversely, argon laser catheters might benefit from sequential firing of a loosely packed array of separated fibers that can be positioned at a greater distance from the catheter tip owing to a more favorable operating range. Again, complexities of catheter design emphasize the importance of an integrated system approach; laser-fiberoptic selection, guidance and control, and catheter delivery system are all interdependent.

GUIDANCE AND CONTROL SYSTEMS

The newest area of development in laser angioplasty delivery systems involves the use of techniques to sample or interrogate proposed target sites to control subsequent laser plaque ablation. Sophisticated guidance and control components within laser catheter systems capable of reliable in vivo plaque recognition may be necessary for safe and efficacious laser atheroma microablation. These "smart" catheters must provide automatic control of rapid pulsed laser activation but must also ensure almost immediate operator feedback, which is imperative for operator override decision making. Lastly, the technique chosen for plaque recognition must be highly sensitive and reliable.

Standard fluoroscopic and angiographic imaging modalities have been the mainstay of present balloon angioplasty procedures. However, early animal and human studies[5-7, 18, 19] have suggested that two-dimensional roentgenographic imaging may not be reliable enough to prevent the possibility of vessel wall perforation during laser angioplasty. Stereoscopic or compound-plane angiography may improve lesion recognition in the future but still is limited to providing a negative image of residual lumen contours. New methods of in vivo plaque recognition currently under investigation include the following: (1) direct fiberoptic visualization (angioscopy); (2) the administration of exogenous fluorescent chromophores that are preferentially sequestered in atheroma[23, 24]; (3) the use of miniature high-frequency ultrasonic crystals encircling the catheter tip to acquire spatial and compositional data; and (4) several spectroscopic techniques, including absorption spectroscopy,[25, 26] infrared spectroscopy, fluorescence spectroscopy, Raman spectroscopy, and photoacoustic spectral analysis. Most of the aforementioned techniques are either speculative or are in embryonic stages of development without substantive published data. However, there is a growing body of knowledge concerning angioscopy and fluorescence spectroscopy worthy of critical review.

Angioscopy

Over the past five years, ultrathin fiberoptic catheters, or angioscopes, have been fabricated by several industry sources and have been used by numerous investigators to study the coronary and peripheral arteries in animals and in humans.[27-31] These devices are flexible, range from 1.0 to 3.7 mm OD, and contain an optical imaging component (coherent bundle of 2,000 to 12,000 fibers), adjacent or circumferential illumination fibers, and a variety of multifunctional working channels. Thus far, angioscopy has been principally used as an investigational tool to examine arterial pathology intraoperatively.[28-31] In the largest series, at the time of coronary artery bypass graft surgery, direct visualization of vascular anatomy using angioscopes has been responsible for a change in the surgical procedure in 26% of patients studied[28] and has helped to characterize the underlying pathophysiology of stable and unstable ischemic chest pain syndromes.[31]

Despite the potential diagnostic and investigational value of angioscopy, there are considerable doubts that high-resolution angioscopy can be incorporated within a multifunctional catheter delivery system for laser angioplasty. Currently, angioscopy must be performed in a bloodless field, which requires both interruption of antegrade blood flow and high-pressure crystalloid infusions to prevent retrograde blood flow from obscuring the field of view. During percutaneous examinations, an inflatable balloon near the catheter tip has been used to occlude the vessel, which prevents antegrade flow, and one of the working channels serves as the infusion port. Catheter bulk and stiffness constraints render it unlikely that a single catheter could accommodate present imaging fiber bundles, illumination fibers, and a flushing channel as well as a laser fiberoptic and perhaps a guide-wire channel for steerability. Nevertheless, even if small, flexible laser-angioscopy catheters could be developed, geometric distortion and nonlinear magnification of the high-resolution images obtained may make rapid and accurate operator interpretation too problematic for laser angioplasty. Until more compact and less complex angioscopy instruments become available, it is unlikely that this guidance and control technique will be a useful adjunct to laser delivery systems.

Fluorescence Spectroscopy

Recently, fluorescence emission spectroscopy has been used in biomedical applications to identify pathologic tissues.[32-34] Moreover, there are now ample data to indicate that fluorescence spectroscopy can reliably differentiate atheroma from surrounding normal arterial wall.[35-38] Analysis of arterial surface fluorescence using quantitative spectral profiles[35-37] and video fluorescence imaging[38] has demonstrated that fluorescence intensity is diminished and spectral characteristics are altered in necropsy specimens of atherosclerotic aorta compared with contiguous normal tissue (Fig 4–6). Importantly, there are also

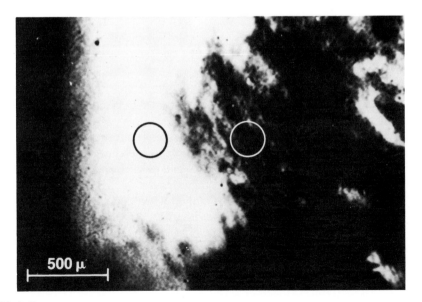

FIG 4–6.
A digitized video fluorescence image using blue light excitation of a fibrous atheroma showing marked contrast differences between normal sites *(black circle)* and diseased sites *(white circle)* in the same frame.

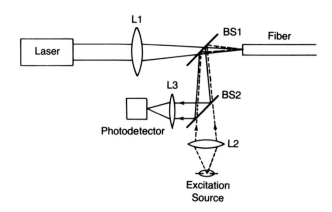

FIG 4–7.
A prototype laser angioplasty fluorescence detection system. Light from an excitation source *(dashed lines)* is focused by a lens (L2) through beam splitters (BS1 and BS2) onto a common fiber, and fluorescence emissions *(solid lines)* are directed back through the same beam splitters to another lens (L3) and onto a photodetector. A laser for ablation is also focused by a lens (L1) through a beam splitter (BS1) onto the same fiber.

data that suggest that surface arterial fluorescence returns to normal after laser atheroma plaque ablation.[39]

The use of fluorescence diagnostics offers intriguing possibilities for the fabrication of a guidance and control unit as a component of a multifunctional laser angioplasty device. Utilizing short pulsed lasers for tissue ablation, there is ample time to excite potential target sites with low-energy monochromatic light and collect fluorescence emissions for compositional analysis, which in turn can be used to activate the laser source for plaque removal. Catheter bulk concerns become less critical since the excitation light, the surface fluorescence emissions, and the laser light for tissue ablation can all be delivered using the same optical fibers employing combinations of beam splitters and dichroic lenses (Fig 4–7). Furthermore, multifiber catheters can be constructed in which individual fibers are responsible for fluorescence plaque identification and subsequent laser ablation for a given tissue zone, providing the capability of selective topographic atheroma vaporization.

Although preliminary data have provided an impetus for continued work on a fluorescence-based multifunctional laser delivery system, the in vivo feasibility of such a device is still speculative. Important design questions remain unanswered and include the following: (1) the reliability of fluorescence detection systems in a blood-filled operating field; (2) the necessity for fiber-target contact for accurate surface fluorescence analysis; (3) the importance of variable-composition atheroma in distinguishing all plaque structures from normal tissue; (4) the alterations in fluorescence emissions associated with laser-induced thermal tissue changes; and (5) the plausibility of shared fibers for target recognition and tissue ablation.

CONCLUSIONS

Laser angioplasty offers great promise as a future catheter-based therapeutic modality in patients with symptomatic peripheral and coronary artery disease. Atherosclerotic plaque ablation may improve on current balloon angioplasty techniques by enabling arterial recanalization in specific anatomic situations, including short and long segments of total obstructions, long segments of diffuse subtotal narrowings, and "hard" lesions that cannot be dilated by mechanical barotrauma. The goal of laser angioplasty is to accomplish atheroma ablation without damaging surrounding normal artery wall or causing inadvertent transmural perforation. The realization of this goal is a formidable engineering task and will demand meticulous adherence to design concepts and adoption of an integrated approach combining laser-fiberoptic selection, multifunctional catheter fabrication, and development of reliable guidance and control systems.

Moreover, seemingly functional systems must be subjected to rigorous, unbiased evaluations in vitro and in animal experiments before human clinical trials. Once safety and efficacy of a system are assured, cautious controlled human studies are indicated, first in patients with peripheral vascular disease, and only later in patients with coronary artery disease. During each phase of the process, data generated will help to modify design concepts, leading to the gradual evolution of valid techniques for clinical use.

REFERENCES

1. Gruntzig AR, Senning A, Sigenthaler WE: Nonoperative dilatation of coronary artery stenoses: Percutaneous transluminal angioplasty. *N Engl J Med* 1979; 301:61–68.
2. Abela GS, Normann SJ, Cohen DM, et al: Laser recanalization off occluded atherosclerotic arteries in vivo and in vitro. *Circulation* 1985; 71:403–411.
3. Crea F, Fenech A, Smith W, et al: Laser recanalization of acutely thrombosed coronary arteries in live dogs: Early results. *J Am Coll Cardiol* 1985; 6:1052–1056.
4. Crea F, Abela GS, Fenech A, et al: Transluminal laser irradiation of coronary arteries in live dogs: An angiographic and morphologic study of acute effects. *Am J Cardiol* 1986; 57:171–174.
5. Ginsburg R, Wexler L, Mitchell RS, et al: Percutaneous transluminal laser angioplasty for treatment of peripheral vascular disease: Clinical response with 16 patients. *Radiology* 1985; 156:619–624.
6. Choy DSJ, Stertzer SH, Myler RK, et al: Human coronary laser recanalization. *Clin Cardiol* 1984; 7:377–381.
7. Abela GS, Seeger JM, Barbieri E, et al: Laser angioplasty with angioscopic guidance in humans. *J Am Coll Cardiol* 1986; 8:184–192.
8. Meyers SM, Bonner RF, Rodrigues MM, et al: Phototransection of vitreal membranes with the carbon dioxide laser in rabbits. *Ophthalmology* 1983; 90:563–568.
9. Grundfest WS, Litvack F, Forrester JS, et al: Laser ablation of human atherosclerotic plaque without adjacent tissue injury. *J Am Coll Cardiol* 1985; 5:929–933.

10. Deckelbaum LI, Isner JM, Donaldson RF, et al: Use of pulsed energy delivery to minimize tissue injury resulting from carbon dioxide laser irradiation of cardiovascular tissues. *J Am Coll Cardiol* 1986; 7:898–908.

11. Linsker R, Srinivasan R, Wynne JJ, et al: Far-ultraviolet laser ablation of atherosclerotic lesions. *Lasers Med Biol* 1984; 4:201–206.

12. Bonner RF, Meyers SM, Gaasterland DE: Threshold for retinal damage associated with the use of high-power neodynium:YAG lasers in the vitreous. *Am J Ophthalmol* 1983; 96:153–159.

13. Deckelbaum LI, Isner JM, Donaldson RF, et al: Reduction of laser-induced pathologic tissue injury using pulsed energy delivery. *Am J Cardiol* 1985; 56:662–667.

14. Abela GS, Normann S, Cohen D, et al: Effects of carbon dioxide, Nd:YAG, and argon laser radiation on coronary atheromatous plaques. *Am J Cardiol* 1982; 50:1199–1205.

15. Choy DSJ, Stertzer SH, Rotterdam HZ, et al: Laser coronary angioplasty: Experience with nine cadaver hearts. *Am J Cardiol* 1982; 50:1209–1211.

16. Anderson HV, Zaatari GS, Roubin GS, et al: Steerable fiberoptic catheter delivery of laser energy in atherosclerotic rabbits. *Am Heart J* 1986; 111:1065–1072.

17. Lee G, Chan MC, Ikeda RM, et al: Applicability of laser to assist coronary balloon angioplasty. *Am Heart J* 1985; 110:1233–1236.

18. Leon MB, Smith PD, Lu DY, et al: In vivo excimer laser angioplasty: Design criteria and preliminary animal results, abstracted. *Circulation* 1986; 74(suppl 2):8.

19. Sanborn TA, Faxon DP, Haudenschild CC, et al: Experimental angioplasty: Circumferential distribution of laser thermal energy with a laser probe. *J Am Coll Cardiol* 1985; 5:934–938.

20. Cumberland DC, Tayler DI, Welsh CL, et al: Percutaneous laser thermal angioplasty: Initial clinical resultss with a laser probe in total peripheral artery occlusions. *Lancet* 1986; 2:1457–1459.

21. Lu DY, Leon MB, Bowman RL: Electrical thermal angioplasty in an atherosclerotic rabbit model, abstracted. *Circulation* 1986; 74(suppl 2):8.

22. Cothren RM, Hayes GB, Kramer JR, et al: A multifiber catheter with an optical shield for laser angiosurgery. *Lasers Life Sci* 1987; 1:1–12.

23. Spears JR, Serur J, Shropstire D, et al: Fluorescence of experimental atheromatous plaques with hematoporphyrin derivative. *J Clin Invest* 1983; 71:395–399.

24. Murphy-Chutorian D, Kosek J, Mok W, et al: Selective absorption of ultraviolet laser energy by human atherosclerotic plaque treated with tetracycline. *Am J Cardiol* 1985; 55:1293–1297.

25. Prince MR, Deutsch TF, Mathews-Roth MM, et al: Preferential light absorption in atheromas in vitro: Implications for laser angioplasty. *J Clin Invest* 1986; 78:295–302.

26. Underhill DJ, Heaney JB, Smith PD, et al: Spectroscopic analysis of human aorta as an aid in laser selection for angioplasty, abstracted. *Circulation* 1985; 72(suppl 3):401.

27. Spears JR, Spokojny AM, Marais HJ: Coronary angioscopy during cardiac catheterization. *J Am Coll Cardiol* 1985; 6:93–97.

28. Underhill DJ, Smith PD, Leon MB, et al: High resolution angioscopy: Feasibility, limitations, and design considerations for laser coronary angioplasty. *Surg Forum* 1985; 36:299–301.

29. Grundfest WS, Litvack F, Sherman CT: Delineation of peripheral and coronary detail by intraoperative angioscopy. *Ann Surg* 1984; 202:394–400.

30. Litvack F, Grundfest WS, Lee ME, et al: Angioscopic visualization of blood vessel interior in animals and humans. *Clin Cardiol* 1985; 8:65–70.
31. Sherman CT, Litvack F, Grundfest W, et al: Coronary angioscopy in patients with unstable angina pectoris. *N Engl J Med* 1986; 315:913–919.
32. Alfano RR, Tata DD, Cordero J, et al: Laser induced fluorescence spectroscopy from native cancerous and normal tissue. *IEEE J Quantum Electron* 1984; 20:1507–1511.
33. Alfano RR, Lam W, Zarrabi H, et al: Human teeth with and without caries studied by laser scattering fluorescence and absorption spectroscopy. *IEEE J Quantum Electron* 1984; 20:1512–1516.
34. Giordano PA, Prosperi E, Bottiroli G: Primary fluorescence of rat muscle after CO_2 laser thermal injury. *Lasers Surg Med* 1984; 4:274–278.
35. Kittrell C, Willett RL, Santos-Pacheo C, et al: Diagnosis of fibrous arterial atherosclerosis using fluorescence. *Appl Optics* 1985; 24:2280–2281.
36. Deckelbaum LI, Lam JK, Cabin HS, et al: Discrimination of normal and atherosclerotic aorta by laser-induced fluorescence, abstracted. *Clin Res* 1986; 34:292.
37. Sartori M, Henry PD, Roberts R: Estimation of arterial wall thickness and detection of atherosclerosis by laser induced argon fluorescence, abstracted. *J Am Coll Cardiol* 1986; 7:207.
38. Lu DY, Leon MB, Smith PD, et al: Atherosclerotic plaque identification using surface fluorescence, abstracted. *Clin Res* 1986; 34:630.
39. Leon MB, Lu DY, Smith PD, et al: Arterial surface fluorescence becomes normal after laser atheroma ablation, abstracted. *Circulation* 1986; 74:II–334.

5

Overview of Laser Applications in the Treatment of Cardiovascular Disease

Thomas L. Robertson, M.D.

Empirical studies of the effects of laser energy on cardiovascular tissues have demonstrated the potential for a variety of therapeutic advances. These include angioplasty, endarterectomy, repair of aneurysms and arterial dissections, venous valvectomy, sealing of vascular anastomoses, transmyocardial neovascularization, myectomy, endocardiectomy, valvuloplasty, interruption of abnormally functioning conduction pathways, ablation of arrhythmogenic foci, and retardation or reversal of atherosclerosis.

The variety and precision of energetic interventions and observational capabilities evolving from laser technology have led to rapid expansion of knowledge in the physical sciences and appreciation of unusual potential in fundamental and applied biomedical research.[1] Lasers now available or in development can produce light energy across much of the electromagnetic spectrum from the far-infrared through the visible and ultraviolet ranges into the x-ray region, from microwatt to terawatt power levels, and from pulse transients of only a few femtoseconds to continuous irradiation.

The utility of lasers in fundamental cardiovascular research has been established. Berns et al.[2] at the University of California in Irvine, using an instrument that incorporates a fine and precise laser irradiating capability through a microscope with computer vision and control, have demonstrated the functional significance of subcellular organelles by sharply localized ablations. For example, ablation of the ribosomal gene area in the X chromosome of cultured cells results in reduced synthesis of ribosomal proteins. This functional deficit is transmitted to subsequent cell generations. In another laser technologic application, Lakatta et al.[3] have used backscattered, laser-induced fluorescence in beating hearts to study the role of calcium ions released from sarcoplasmic reticulum. This group is currently using this methodology to determine the role of calcium cycling in the generation of late systolic afterpotentials during ischemia and reperfusion.

Progress toward clinical applications has been impeded by technical difficulties and, importantly, by lack of specific information about laser energy interaction with cardiovascular tissues. It has become apparent that the effects of laser energy on tissue differ widely according to lasing parameters and the specific characteristics of the tissue and surrounding medium.[4] To evaluate adequately the potential uses of laser technology for treatment of cardiovascular disease, systematic studies are needed to observe short- and long-term tissue effects according to laser wavelength, energy level, and timing characteristics with consideration of the modulating effects of the surrounding medium.

NATURE OF LASER EFFECTS ON TISSUE

The physical properties of tissue and surrounding medium (blood, interstitial fluid, and irrigating solutions) determine focus, reflection, and scattering of laser energy as well as conduction of resultant thermal energy away from the site of laser-tissue interaction. Thus, the operating characteristics of the laser and optical and other properties of the tissue and surrounding medium interact to determine the depth of penetration, the volume of tissue affected, and the induced physical changes.

Whereas physical changes have been attributed usually to thermal effects (dehydration, coagulation, charring, and gasification), at high energy and short pulse duration, photochemical mechanisms may result in disruption of chemical bonds. Laser-induced, high-energy plasma formation can be used to disintegrate tissue in a controlled fashion. Also, tissue effects may be modulated by the presence of chromophores. At low power, clinically relevant differences in fluorescence may be induced, and this may prove to be useful diagnostically and as a guide to therapy. In addition, other therapeutically useful tissue effects may be mediated by other mechanisms.

VARIETY OF LASERS

Of the numerous lasers that are available from commercial suppliers, a number are being evaluated for cardiovascular applications. These include carbon dioxide (CO_2), erbium:yttrium-aluminum-garnet (YAG), carbon monoxide, neodymium (Nd):YAG, alexandrite, argon ion, tunable dye, krypton ion, copper vapor, gold vapor, and excimer lasers. Other lasers are in development, such as the free-electron lasers, which will provide wavelengths not currently available with other lasers. Certain CO_2, Nd:YAG, and argon ion lasers have become available for ophthalmologic, dermatologic, or general surgical indications, and these have been evaluated most extensively for potential cardiovascular applications.[5-8] However, the lasing characteristics needed for specific cardiovascular applications may require developmental initiative. For example, Forrester et al.[9] have been able to ablate cardiovascular tissue in vivo in a reproducible, controlled fashion using pulsed ultraviolet laser energy from a specially constructed xenon chloride excimer laser, which is conducted through a proprietary optical fiber, whereas other investigative teams have had difficulty reproducing similar results with commercially available devices.

ANGIOPLASTY

Several approaches to percutaneous angioplasty have been investigated using a variety of laser energy sources and optical fibers to conduct the laser energy to obstructing arterial lesions. Several investigative teams have attempted to use argon ion or Nd:YAG laser energy conducted through an optical fiber, introduced through guiding catheters, to remove arterial obstructions. Ginsberg et al.[10] reported improvement in blood flow in peripheral arteries following penetration of obstructing atherosclerotic plaques, which could then be dilated with conventional balloon angioplasty technique. Because perforation of the arterial wall or thrombosis occurred in several patients, these investigators concluded that further laboratory investigation and laser-catheter system development were needed.

Optical Fibers

Commercially available optical fibers transmit the near-infrared and visible wavelengths with relatively little energy loss and have been used intravascularly with Nd:YAG and argon ion lasers in animal and clinical experimental studies, as noted above. With bare optical fibers, perforation of the arterial wall has been a problem attributed to both mechanical and thermal mechanisms; stiffness of some optical fibers appears to be a factor in mechanical perforation. Furthermore, clot and debris may accumulate on the fiber tip during intravascular laser irradiation. This may result in "burn back" (damage to the distal end of the fiber) or in bonding of the fiber to the arterial wall; the former interrupts transmission of laser energy from the distal end of the fiber, and the latter results in detachment of variable amounts of arterial intima and media when the fiber is withdrawn. Optical fibers are under development which meet flexibility and peak power requirements for transmission of pulsed ultraviolet and mid-infrared laser energy in vivo.

Thermal Probes

The problems with the distal ends of optical fibers have been approached in several ways. Two general types of metal caps have been attached to the ends of optical fibers and used as thermal probes to open arterial obstructions. One is solid and another is open at the end. Both are heated rapidly by laser energy conducted through the optical fibers and are operated in the 200 to 400° C range to vaporize or melt atheromatous arterial obstructions. Thermal probes with open tips provide egress of the laser beam to irradiate arterial obstruction distal to the catheter tip. These systems are being evaluated as means to create larger channels than result with the solid metal-tipped probes.[11]

Metal-tipped laser catheter systems have been used in over 200 peripheral arterial angioplasties and over a dozen coronary angioplasties; thermal probes have been used to penetrate tight stenoses or total occlusions, including cases with long occlusions. The resulting channels, though small, allow placement of conventional balloon angioplasty catheters, which are then used in the conventional way to dilate obstructions. Investigators evaluating thermal probes are attempting to determine the following: (1) success of angioplasty in cases with advanced disease not suitable for conventional balloon angioplasty, including frequency of improved perfusion, failure to penetrate obstructions, and perforation and thrombosis rates; (2) long-term results, including clinical outcome and frequency of continued patency and recurrent stenosis.

Preliminary results by Abela et al.[12] and Sanborn et al.[13] in the United States and by Cumberland et al.[14] in England suggest that thermal probes may offer advantages for some patients. There is inadequate information to evaluate the long-term outcome of thermal injury to the arterial wall. There are preliminary indications that successful opening and restenosis rates may favor thermal probe–initiated angioplasty over conventional balloon catheter–initiated angioplasty in patients with peripheral vascular disease.[15] It may be speculated that myointimal proliferation or recurrent atherosclerosis at the site of angioplasty may be retarded by thermal injury, but the potential for late scar formation or thrombosis requires further evaluation.

Other Contact Probes

Fourrier et al.[16] in France have developed a catheter system that uses an Nd:YAG laser coupled to an optical fiber, which in turn is coupled to a sapphire contact tip. With this experimental system, relatively long obstructions in peripheral arteries in a few patients have been recanalized. Other contact-tip laser-catheter systems are also under development.

An optical shield is under development by Cothren et al. at the Massachusetts Institute of Technology, and Kramer et al. at the Cleveland Clinic Foundation.[17] This approach may obviate some of the disadvantages encountered with bare optical fibers and with metal-tipped catheters. An optically clear glass cap is attached to the end of a catheter that incorporates an array of optical fibers, which are fixed in relation to the optical shield so that overlapping laser beams emitted from the fibers irradiate distally in a controlled fashion. This catheter system is being developed with the capability for machine discrimination of laser-induced fluorescence patterns to differentiate atheroma from normal arterial-wall tissue. In operation, the optical shield at the end of the catheter would be pressed against an obstructing atheroma. A low-power laser beam would be used to induce fluorescence, and a distinctive pattern typical of atheroma would trigger irradiation through the optical fibers that are aimed at the atheroma. Cessation of the typical fluorescence and/or sensing of normal arterial wall tissue would signal termination of irradiation through the relevant optical fibers. Optical fibers not focused on tissue producing the laser fluorescence signal typical of atheroma would not be energized. This *intelligent* catheter system may be adapted for use with a variety of laser fiberoptic configurations according to future developments.

Pulsed Laser Catheter Systems

To obviate thermal injury to arterial tissue, several investigative teams have evaluated pulsed lasers with operating parameters that result in little or no evidence of residual injury to the arterial wall.[18–20] Laboratory experiments with infrared, visible light, and ultraviolet laser energy delivered in 10 to 100-nsec pulses have been reported in which atherosclerotic plaque was ablated with minimal injury to the remaining tissue. Katzir et al.[21] and Sartori et al.[22] have investigated the use of pulsed Nd:YAG and excimer lasers to produce clean ablation. With appropriate operating parameters, comparable smooth ablation was obtained with minimal thermal injury to the remaining arterial wall. These experimental results indicate that pulsed laser energy at a variety of wavelengths may be used to remove pathologic cardiovascular tissue, including calcified atherosclerotic tissue, without significant residual tissue injury.

The mechanism responsible for clean ablation is disputed. The photoproducts resulting from such ablation have been described, on the one hand, as characteristic of thermal processes but, on the other hand, as characteristic of photochemical reactions. Calmettes and Berns[23] have published results indicating that, under certain conditions, multiphoton processes occur. Depending on the experimental conditions, the products of such ablation may include particles on the order of many microns in size.[24]

An impediment to the use of pulsed laser energy for percutaneous angioplasty is the need for optical fibers that can deliver pulsed laser energy sufficient for ablation without fiber breakdown in vivo. Forrester et al.[9] have reported progress in the development of an experimental optical fiber that conducts sufficient energy from a xenon chloride excimer laser for ablation of atherosclerotic plaque and other tissues. There is preliminary evidence of clean ablation using erbium:YAG laser energy in the mid-infrared region of the electromagnetic spectrum, which is conducted through a zirconium fluoride fiberoptic waveguide.[25]

ENDARTERECTOMY

Laser endarterectomy has been evaluated in experimental animals and, to a limited extent, in patients at open surgery. Eugene et al.[26–28] compared endarterectomy performed with CO_2, Nd:YAG, and argon ion lasers to remove atherosclerotic intima in experimental studies. Results with the argon laser were superior as to ease of performance, smoothness of the resulting luminal surfaces, adherence of remaining intima and media, damage to the arterial wall, and healing characteristics. Using a hand-held CO_2 laser, Livesay et al.,[29] in a preliminary report, indicated successful short-term results with distal endarterectomy in coronary artery revascularization procedures in a small series of patients.

ABLATION OF MYOCARDIUM

Myotomy, Myectomy, and Transmyocardial Neovascularization

Experimental studies and early clinical experiments have demonstrated the feasibility of removing or altering myocardial tissue for therapeutic objectives. Isner and Clarke[30] used an argon laser to perform myotomy and myectomy in a patient with asymmetric septal hypertrophy with resulting clinical improvement in left ventricular outlet obstruction. Preliminary work by Mirhoseini and Clayton[31] in the United States and investigators in Japan and the Soviet Union suggests that neovascularization of ischemic myocardial tissue may follow creation of channels by transmyocardial laser irradiation. Under certain conditions these new channels were reported to endothelialize and provide for the flow of blood directly from the left ventricle. These results have not been confirmed by other investigators in the United States.

Arrhythmia Control: Photoablation and Endocardiectomy

Several investigative teams have evaluated CO_2, Nd:YAG, and argon laser energy to ablate abnormally functioning cardiac conduction tissue or arrhythmogenic foci.[32–36] Experiments with both percutaneous and open surgical approaches suggest that laser ablation may be performed in a more precise manner than with conventional techniques. The potential for percutaneous approaches has generated interest among investigators, and the development of catheter systems that would incorporate electrophysiologic, angioscopic, and laser irradiating capabilities.

VALVULOPLASTY

In preliminary experimental work, Isner and Clarke[37] have found that calcific deposits on otherwise normal-appearing valves may be ablated without significant damage to the underlying valvular structures. Such an approach, if further developed, could provide an alternative to valve replacement in some patients. Ultimately, it may be possible to develop a system for safe percutaneous removal of atherosclerotic and calcific accretions from cardiac valves.

VASCULAR REPAIR

Construction of Anastomoses

Conventional surgical anastomoses may be complicated by bleeding or thrombosis and by late closure due to granuloma formation, scarring, myointimal hyperplasia, or atherosclerosis. To improve clinical outcome, several investigators have evaluated CO_2, Nd:YAG, and argon ion lasers for a variety of anastomoses.[38-41] Early results suggest that tissue sealing and fusion at anastomotic sites may be accomplished with disparate laser parameters. Arteriovenous anastomoses in experimental animals produced with the argon ion laser have compared favorably with conventional technique as to increased anastomotic strength, thrombogenicity, and healing characteristics. In addition to laser wavelength, results may depend also on the laser energy delivery system, the technical details of instrument and tissue manipulation, and the size and specific characteristics of the vessels to be fused and sealed.

Aneurysm Repair

Progress has been made in the development of approaches to repairing arterial aneurysms in experimental animals. In the animal model developed by O'Reilly et al.,[42] aneurysm cavities have been partially obliterated by inducing clot formation and local tissue injury, which was followed by fibrosis and reendothelialization of the luminal surface.

Arterial dissection occurs spontaneously in acute aortic dissection or iatrogenically following angioplasty. Animal experiments have demonstrated the feasibility of fusing dissected intima to the media by first reapproximating the dissected tissue planes with a special balloon angioplasty catheter and then irradiating through the balloon with an Nd:YAG laser.[43-45] This approach may compete with other percutaneous catheter techniques under development for placement of vascular stents in dissected segments of artery.

CHROMOPHORES

Following the work of Spears et al.[46] in which hematoporphyrin derivative was shown to have affinity for atherosclerotic tissue, considerable interest has focused on the use of dyes that are preferentially absorbed by atherosclerotic tissue and absorb light at wavelengths that are minimally absorbed by normal tissue. Tetracycline has been evaluated by several investigators because of its staining characteristics and absorption peaks at wavelengths generated by the argon laser. Abela et al.[47] reported selective ablation of atherosclerotic lesions in an animal model following tetracycline staining and argon laser irradiation. In this controlled study, evidence of regression was observed in both the control and tetracycline-treated groups, but the degree of regression was substantially greater in the tetracycline-stained vessels.

Prince et al.[48] reported the ablation of human atherosclerotic tissue with minimal injury to adjacent normal arterial intima when a tunable dye laser at low power was used at a wavelength that was preferentially absorbed by naturally occurring carotenoids that accumulate preferentially within atherosclerotic plaque. These encouraging experiments suggest that endogenous or exogenous chromophores that concentrate preferentially in atheroma may provide the means for selective ablation or for inducing regression of atherosclerotic tissue with minimal or no injury to normal arterial wall.

REGRESSION OF ATHEROSCLEROSIS

Gerrity et al.[49] observed rapid healing, intimal fibrous scarring, but no indication of accelerated atherosclerotic response at 8 weeks following low-energy CO_2 laser removal of atherosclerotic plaques in hyperlipemic swine. In hypercholesterolemic, atherosclerotic rhesus monkeys, Abela et al.[50] showed evidence consistent with regression of atherosclerotic plaque in areas adjacent to iliofemoral arterial sites that had been ablated 7 to 60 days earlier by argon ion laser irradiation delivered through an optical fiber. Thus, evidence of regression or reduced bulk of atherosclerotic tissue has followed subablative[49, 50] and low-power laser radiation as noted above.[47] The mechanism of these regressive changes is unclear. Regression following laser irradiation near ablative levels suggests a thermal effect; however, the low-power experiment suggests a mechanism other than response to thermal injury. If laser-induced regression or interruption of progression of atherosclerosis can be demonstrated as a long-term effect, important new therapeutic advantages may be realized with percutaneous angioplasty and for open surgical endarterectomy and anastomosis in revascularization procedures.

SUMMARY

Laboratory and preliminary clinical investigations have demonstrated that the use of lasers in the treatment of a number of cardiovascular problems is feasible. A variety of approaches is being studied with an increasing number of laser systems. Ideal operating parameters for specific applications are yet to be determined. Recent progress suggests that therapeutic advances will be realized in anastomotic sealing, endarterectomy, percutaneous removal of arterial obstruction, regression of atherosclerosis, open surgical percutaneous ablation of arrhythmogenic foci and abnormal conduction pathways, and other cardiovascular applications.

REFERENCES

1. Hochstrasser RM, Carey KJ: Lasers in biology. *Laser Focus/Electro-opt* 1985; 21:100–118.
2. Berns MW, Aist J, Edwards J, et al: Laser microsurgery in cell and developmental biology. *Science* 1981; 213:505–513.
3. Lakatta EG, Capogrossi C, Kort AA, et al: Spontaneous myocardial calcium oscillations: Overview with emphasis on ryanadine and caffeine. *Fed Proc* 1985; 2977–2983.
4. Regan JD, Parrish JA: *The Science of Photomedicine.* New York, Plenum Publishing Corp, 1982.
5. Abela GS, Normann S, Cohen D, et al: Effects of carbon dioxide, Nd:YAG, and argon laser radiation on coronary atheromatous plaques. *Am J Cardiol* 1982; 50:1199–1205.
6. Isner JM, Clarke RH: The current status of lasers in the treatment of cardiovascular disease. *IEEE J Quantum Electronics* 1984; 20:1406–1420.
7. Gerschwind HJ, Boussignac G, Teisseire B, et al: Conditions for effective Nd:YAG laser angioplasty. *Br Heart J* 1984; 52:484–489.
8. Macrue R, Martins JRM, Tupinamba AS: Possibilidades terapeuticas do raio laser em atromas. *Arq Bras Cardiol* 1980; 35:9–12.
9. Forrester JS, Litvack F, Grundfest WS: Laser angioplasty and cardiovascular disease. *Am J Cardiol* 1986; 57:990–992.
10. Ginsberg R, Wexler L, Mitchell RS, et al: Percutaneous transluminal laser angioplasty for treatment of peripheral vascular disease: Clinical experience with 16 patients. *Radiology* 1985; 156:619–624.
11. Abela GS, Barbieri E, Roxey T, et al: A method of quantitative plaque ablation using power-time matrix laser application, abstracted. *Circulation* 1986; 74(suppl 2):6.
12. Abela GS, Seeger JM, Barbieri E, et al: Laser recanalization under angioscopic guidance in humans. *J Am Coll Cardiol* 1986; 8:182–194.
13. Sanborn TA, Greenfield AJ, Guben JK, et al: Human percutaneous and intraoperative laser thermal angioplasty—Initial clinical results as an adjunct to balloon angioplasty. *J Vasc Surg* 1987; 5:183–190.
14. Cumberland DC, Sanborn TA, Taylor DI, et al: Percutaneous laser thermal angioplasty—Initial clinical results with a laserprobe in total peripheral artery occlusions. *Lancet* 1986; 1:1457–1459.
15. Sanborn TA, Faxon DP, Christian C, et al: Laser thermal angioplasty: Reduced restenosis compared to balloon angioplasty, abstracted. *Circulation* 1986; 74(suppl 2):6.
16. Fourrier JL, Marache P, Brunetaud J, et al: Laser recanalization of peripheral arteries by contact sapphire in man, abstracted. *Circulation* 1986; 74(suppl 2):204.
17. Cothren RM, Hayes GB, Cramer JR, et al: A multifiber catheter with an optical shield for laser angiosurgery. *Lasers Life Sci* 1987; 1:1–12.

18. Grundfest WS, Litvack F, Forrester JS, et al: Laser ablation of human atherosclerotic plaque without adjacent tissue injury. *J Am Coll Cardiol* 1985; 5:929–933.

19. Deckelbaum LI, Isner JM, Donaldson RF, et al: Use of pulsed energy delivery to minimize tissue injury resulting from carbon dioxide laser irradiation of cardiovascular tissues. *J Am Coll Cardiol* 1986; 7:898–908.

20. Linsker R, Srinivasan R, Wynne JJ, et al: Far-ultraviolet laser ablation of atherosclerotic lesions. *Lasers Med Biol* 1984; 4:201–206.

21. Katzir A, Isner JM, Clarke RH, et al: Development of an infrared fiber radiometer for non-contact temperature monitoring during laser irradiation: Initial measurements regarding mechanism of ablation, abstracted. *Circulation* 1986; 74(suppl 2):497.

22. Sartori MP, Henry PD, Sauerbrey RA, et al: Tissue interaction and measurement of ablation rates with UV and visible lasers in canine and human arteries. *Lasers Surg Med,* in press.

23. Calmettes PP, Berns MW: Laser induced multiphoton processes in living cells. *Proc Natl Acad Sci USA* 1983; 80:7197–7199.

24. DeJesus ST, Isner JM, Rongione AJ, et al: Embolic potential of cardiovascular laser irradiation. *Proc Soc Photo-Opt Instr Engl* 1986; 713:47–49.

25. Bonner RF, Smith PD, Leon M, et al: A new erbium laser and infrared fiber system for laser angioplasty, abstracted. *Circulation* 1986; 74(suppl 2):361.

26. Eugene J, McColgan SJ, Pollock ME, et al: Experimental arteriosclerosis treated by conventional and laser endarterectomy. *J Surg Med* 1985; 39:31–38.

27. Eugene J, Pollock ME, McColgan SJ, et al: Fiber optic versus direct laser delivery for endarterectomy of experimental atheromas. *Proc Int Soc Opt Eng* 1985; 576:55–58.

28. Eugene J, McColgan SJ, Pollock ME, et al: Experimental arteriosclerosis treated by argon ion and neodymium-YAG laser endarterectomy. *Circulation* 1985; 72(suppl 2):200–206.

29. Livesay JJ, Leachman DR, Hogan PJ, et al: Preliminary report on laser coronary endarterectomy in patients. *Circulation* 1985; 72(suppl 3):302.

30. Isner JM, Clarke RH: Laser myoplasty for hypertrophic cardiomyopathy: In vitro experience in human postmortem hearts and in vivo experience in a canine model (transarterial) and human patients (intraoperative). *Am J Cardiol* 1984; 53:1620–1625.

31. Mirhoseini M, Clayton MM: Revascularization of the heart by laser. *J Microsurg* 1981; 2:253–260.

32. Abela GS, Griffin JC, Hill JA, et al: Transvascular argon laser induced atrial ventricular conduction ablation in dogs, abstracted. *Circulation* 1983; 68(suppl 3):580.

33. Lee BI, Gottdiener JS, Fletcher RD, et al: Transcatheter ablation: Comparison between laser photoablation and electrode shock ablation in the dog. *Circulation* 1985; 71:579–586.

34. Isner JM, Estes NAM, Payne DD, et al: Laser assisted endocardiectomy for refractory ventricular tachyarrythmias: Preliminary intraoperative experience. *Clin Cardiol* 1987; 10:201–204.

35. Svenson RH, Gallagher JJ, Selle JK, et al: Intraoperative laser photoablation of ventricular tachycardia, abstracted. *Circulation* 1986; 74(suppl 2):461.

36. Saksena S, Hussain SM, Gelchinsky I: Successful mapping-guided argon laser ablation of ventricular tachycardia in man. *Circulation* 1986; 74(suppl 2):186.

37. Isner JM, Clarke RH: Laser-assisted debridement of aortic valve calcium. *Am Heart J* 1985; 109:448–452.

38. Schober R, Ulrich F, Sander T, et al: Laser-induced alteration of collagen substructure allows microsurgical tissue welding. *Science* 1986; 232:1421–1422.

39. McCarthy WJ, Hartz RS, Yao JST, et al: Vascular anastomoses with laser energy. *J Vasc Surg* 1986; 3:32–41.

40. Frazier OH, Painvin GA, Morris JM, et al: Laser assisted microvascular anastomoses—Angiographic and anatomopathologic studies on growing microvascular anastomoses—Preliminary report. *Surgery* 1985; 97:585–590.

41. White RA: Technical frontiers for the vascular surgeon: Laser vascular anastomotic welding and angioscopy-assisted intraluminal instrumentation. *J Vasc Surg* 1987; 5:673–680.

42. O'Reilly GV, Forrest MD, Schoene WC, et al: Laser induced thermal coagulation of berry aneurysms: Preliminary experimental experience. Submitted for publication.

43. Hiehle JF Jr, Bourgelais DBC, Shapshay S, et al: Nd:YAG laser fusion of human atheromatous plaque-arterial wall separations in vitro. *Am J Cardiol* 1985; 56:953–957.

44. Serur JR, Sinclair IN, Spokojny AM, et al: Laser balloon angioplasty (LBA): Effect on the carotid lumen in the dog, abstracted. *Circulation* 1985; 72(suppl 3):457.

45. Sanborn TA, Sinclair IN, Serur JR, et al: In vivo laser thermal seal of neointimal dissection after balloon angioplasty in rabbit atherosclerosis, abstracted. *Circulation* 1985; 72(suppl 3):469.

46. Spears JR, Serur J, Shropshire D, et al: Fluorescence of experimental atheromatous plaques with hematoporphyrin derivative. *J Clin Invest* 1983; 71:395–397.

47. Abela GS, Barbieri E, Roxey T, et al: Laser enhanced plaque atherolysis with tetracycline, abstracted. *Circulation* 1986; 72(suppl 2):7.

48. Prince MR, Deutsch TF, Mathews-Roth MM, et al: Preferential light absorption in atheromas in vitro. *J Clin Invest* 1986; 78:295–302.

49. Gerrity RG, Coop FD, Golding AR, et al: Arterial response to laser operation for removal of atherosclerotic plaques. *J Thorac Cardiovasc Surg* 1983; 85:409–421.

50. Abela GS, Crea F, Seeger JE, et al: The healing process in normal canine arteries and in atherosclerotic monkey arteries after transluminal laser irradiation. *Am J Cardiol* 1985; 56:983–988.

6

Laser Thermal Angioplasty

Timothy A. Sanborn, M.D.

Though balloon angioplasty is now a well-accepted alternative to bypass surgery for high-grade obstructive atherosclerotic lesions of the peripheral, renal, and coronary vessels,[1] it still has a number of limitations. Despite a primary success rate that approaches 90% to 95%, the procedure is complicated by a 20% to 40% restenosis rate.[2, 3] In addition, balloon angioplasty is less successful in totally occluded vessels. In coronary arteries, for example, a success rate of only 54% has been reported.[4, 5] As laser energy has been shown to be effective in removing atherosclerotic lesions experimentally[6–13] and clinically,[14–22] it is hypothesized that by removing atherosclerotic obstructions through vaporization of plaque, laser angioplasty may be an effective adjunct or alternative to balloon angioplasty. However, to date the technique has been limited by inadequate delivery systems, resulting in an unacceptably high perforation rate[11, 12, 15, 16] and the creation of small recanalized channels, which result in poor long-term patency.[16]

HISTORICAL PERSPECTIVE

Historically, interest in the use of lasers to vaporize atherosclerotic lesions began with in vitro studies on postmortem specimens. Marcruz et al.[6] were the first to report the use of an argon laser to destroy calcific and noncalcific aortic specimens at various laser exposures, incidence angles, and focal sizes. This was followed by the demonstration by Lee et al.[7] and Abela et al.[8] that argon, neodymium:yttrium-aluminum-garnet (Nd:YAG), and carbon dioxide (CO_2) laser wavelengths could all be used to produce a "wedge" incision in the atherosclerotic coronary artery segments. However, it was not until Choy et al. reported on successful transluminal laser angioplasty using flexible fiberoptic fibers in vivo in animals[9] and in vitro in cadaveric coronary vessels[10] that real interest in the possibility of laser angioplasty developed. In these experimental studies, however, a high incidence of vessel perforation was noted when laser light was emitted from bare fiberoptic fibers positioned using fluoroscopic guidance alone.[11, 12]

INITIAL CLINICAL STUDIES

In the early phase of laser angioplasty investigation, several clinical studies were initiated. Ginsberg et al.[14] were the first to report a case of successful peripheral laser angioplasty in which a 200-μm argon laser fiber was positioned at the end of a balloon catheter and used to recanalize a 95% deep profunda artery stenosis. Subsequently, Ginsberg et al.[15] reported results in 16 patients; the procedure was successful in 8 of 17 (47%) peripheral vessels, with three laser perforations. Later, Choy et al.[16] performed intraoperative human coronary artery laser recanalization with an argon laser in five patients during coronary artery bypass grafting. The procedure was successful in three patients, with one mechanical perforation; however, no recanalizations were patent at follow-up angioplasty longer than three months, owing, in part, to the influence of competition for flow from concurrent bypass grafts. In addition, Geschwind et al.[17] reported successful percutaneous peripheral laser angioplasty using an Nd:YAG laser in three patients; however, clinical or angiographic follow-up was not included in this brief report.

Recently, further clinical advances were made when Livesay et al.[18] reported on intraoperative laser coronary endarterectomy as an adjunct to bypass surgery using a hand-held CO_2 laser device in eight patients. In a total of 16 coronary arteries, follow-up angiography one week after the procedure demonstrated vessel patency in the treated area in 12 of 16 (75%) of the arteries. However, use of this rigid device was limited to 2 to 3 cm from the arteriotomy site; this limitation may preclude widespread clinical application.

Abela et al.,[22] in an ongoing clinical study, used an angioscope to visualize laser recanalization under direct vision during peripheral artery bypass surgery in an attempt to diminish the incidence of vessel perforation. Initial clinical attempts using the angioscope to direct a bare argon fiberoptic fiber were still plagued by perforation in 6 of 13 arteries; however, better results were obtained in later cases performed with a 2-mm laser probe-type device similar to that to be discussed subsequently in this chapter.

Thus, the key issue in clinical laser angioplasty has been the lack of an adequate catheter-delivery system for safe and effective intravascular use. The first laser fiberoptic-catheter system to be developed that shows promise in preliminary animal and clinical trials is the Laserprobe.

THE LASERPROBE

Experimental Results

In the last few years, a novel fiberoptic laser delivery system, the Laserprobe, has been developed (Trimedyne, Inc) in which argon laser energy is converted to heat in a rounded metallic cap at the end of a fiberoptic fiber. Two experimental studies have been performed comparing angiographic and histologic results using this new laser device with those using a bare fiberoptic fiber.[11, 15] Using a rabbit iliac model of atherosclerosis, we were able to compare the results in 24 rabbits randomly assigned to laser angioplasty with either of these two modalities. Both fibers had similar outer (0.9 mm) and core (400 μm) diameters (Fig 6–1). Pulses of 1 W for 1 second's duration were delivered from the tip of the bare fiberoptic fiber, whereas pulses of 6 W for 2 seconds' duration were delivered from the Laserprobe. Angiographic widening of luminal stenoses was seen in 2 of 12 rabbits with the standard fiberoptic system, whereas 8 of 12 rabbits treated with the Laserprobe demonstrated luminal enlargement ($P < .001$). More importantly, perforation of the vessel wall occurred frequently with the fiberoptic fiber (9 of 12 rabbits) as opposed to only one mechanical perforation in 12 rabbits treated with the Laserprobe ($P < .001$). Table 6–1 and Figure 6–2 summarize these experimental results.

Histologic examination of vessels treated with direct laser radiation from the fiberoptic fiber revealed a small, localized laser defect along one side of the vessel wall associated with charring, a gradient of thermal injury, and considerable thrombus formation. In contrast, those vessels treated with the La-

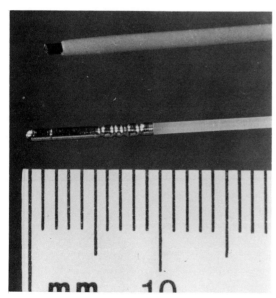

FIG 6–1.
Fiberoptic fibers. A 0.9-mm outer-diameter quartz fiber (400-μm core) inserted in a standard 5 F angiographic catheter *(top)*. A 0.9-mm outer-diameter quartz fiber (400-μm core) with rounded metallic tip secured at the end of the fiber *(bottom)*. (From Sanborn TA, Faxon DP, Haudenschild C, et al: Experimental angioplasty—Circumferential distribution of laser thermal energy with a laser probe. *J Am Coll Cardiol* 1985; 5:934–938. Reproduced by permission.)

TABLE 6–1.

Angiographic Results in 12 Rabbits*†

| | LUMINAL STENOSIS, % | | | | ANGIOGRAPHIC SUCCESS | | PERFORATION | |
| | BEFORE TREATMENT | | AFTER TREATMENT | | | | | |
CASE NO.	FIBEROPTIC FIBER	LASER PROBE	FIBEROPTIC FIBER	LASER PROBE	FIBEROPTIC FIBER	LASER PROBE	FIBEROPTIC FIBER	LASER PROBE
1	90	50	90	0	0	+	+	0
2	50	50	30	30	+	+	0	0
3	50	50	50	30	0	+	0	0
4	30	50	−	50	0	0	+	+
5	90	90	−	90	0	0	+	0
6	70	90	−	90	0	0	0	0
7	90	50	−	50	0	0	+	0
8	50	90	30	0	+	+	+	0
9	70	90	−	30	0	+	+	0
10	90	70	−	0	0	+	+	0
11	40	70	40	0	0	+	+	0
12	50	70	−	0	0	+	+	0
Total or mean ± SD	64 ± 21	68 ± 17‡	. . .	. . .	2	8§	9	1‖

*From Sanborn TA, Faxon DP, Haudenschild C, et al: Experimental angioplasty—Circumferential distribution of laser thermal energy with a laser probe. J Am Coll Cardiol 1985; 5:934–938.
†Reproduced by permission. Plus indicates presence; 0, absence; minus, percent stenosis could not be determined because dye extravasation obscured the lumen.
‡Not significant.
§$P < .01$.
‖$P < .001$.

serprobe showed histologic evidence of thermal injury distributed evenly around the entire luminal circumference (Fig 6–3). The thermal effect produced by the Laserprobe was associated with minimal charring, a gradient of thermal injury, and thinner, flatter thrombus formation (Fig 6–4).

Thus, the Laserprobe was found to alleviate luminal stenosis more effectively with less vessel perforation than a currently available fiberoptic-catheter system. The histologic data suggest that circumferential rather than localized narrowly directed distribution of laser energy may be a factor in these improved results.

Abela et al.[22] have confirmed these results in a smaller series of human coronary artery xenografts in which postmortem human coronary arteries were transplanted into the canine femoral artery and left intact for four weeks. Angiography demonstrated recanalization in all five arteries treated with the Laserprobe and three of five arteries treated with the bare fiber. Only one perforation occurred with the Laserprobe, whereas three perforations occurred with the bare fiberoptic fiber. The larger 1.5-mm Laserprobe was also capable of creating a larger channel in the occluded arterial segment.

Recent follow-up angiographic and histologic studies in our laboratory demonstrated good long-term patency with minimal thrombogenesis and a

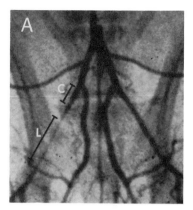
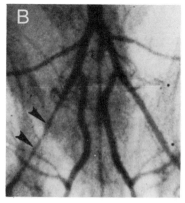

FIG 6–2.
Angiographic example of a Laserprobe angioplasty. **A,** long, tubular, 90% mid-right iliac artery lesion *(L)* relative to a proximal control segment *(C).* **B,** lesion after treatment with two pulses (6 W, 2 seconds), 1 cm apart, resulting in a 30% residual stenosis *(arrowheads).* (From Sanborn TA, Faxon DP, Haudenschild C, et al: Experimental angioplasty—Circumferential distribution of laser thermal energy with a laser probe. *J Am Coll Cardiol* 1985; 5:934–938. Reproduced by permission.)

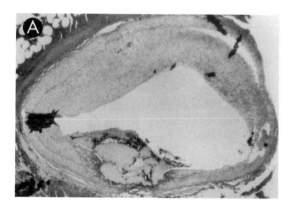

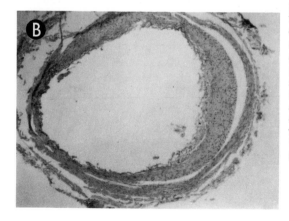

FIG 6–3.
A, example of direct argon laser radiation resulting in a localized defect along one side of the iliac artery wall, which extends through the neointima into the media. A gradient of thermal injury characterized by cell swelling and tissue edema is also noted. In addition, considerable thrombus is present that fills the newly formed laser defect. **B,** example of Laserprobe thermal injury distributed evenly around the entire luminal circumference. Hematoxylin-eosin; × 80. (From Sanborn TA, Faxon DP, Haudenschild C, et al: Experimental angioplasty—Circumferential distribution of laser thermal energy with a laser probe. *J Am Coll Cardiol* 1985; 5:934–938. Reproduced by permission.)

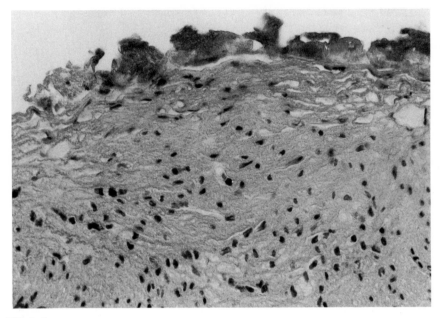

FIG 6–4.
Magnified histologic section of Laserprobe thermal injury demonstrating a thin, flat platelet thrombus and a gradient of thermal injury involving the inner layer of the neointima without damage to the outer layer of the neointima or media (hematoxylin-eosin, × 500). (From Sanborn TA, Faxon DP, Haudenschild C, et al: Experimental angioplasty—Circumferential distribution of laser thermal energy with a laser probe. *J Am Coll Cardiol* 1985; 5:934–938. Reproduced by permission.)

very mild proliferative response to laser thermal angioplasty with a 1.5- to 2.0-mm Laserprobe in the rabbit atherosclerosis model.[23] On histologic examination, reendothelialization of the luminal surface was noted as early as 2 weeks after laser angioplasty. At 4 weeks the neointima was thin with a fibrous cap and minimal fibrocellular proliferation (Fig 6–5).

Clinical Studies

With the described background in experimental animals, we began a clinical trial to determine the safety and efficacy of the Laserprobe in performing percutaneous laser angioplasty as an adjunct to balloon angioplasty in patients with severe peripheral vascular disease.[19] Collaborating vascular radiologists included David C. Cumberland, M.D., and David I. Tayler, M.D., at Northern General Hospital in Sheffield, England, and Alan J. Greenfield, M.D., and Jon K. Guben, M.D., at Boston University Medical Center. The patient population in this study consisted of patients with severe claudication, rest pain, or threatened limb loss who would be candidates for balloon angioplasty or bypass surgery of superficial femoral or popliteal artery stenoses or occlusions.

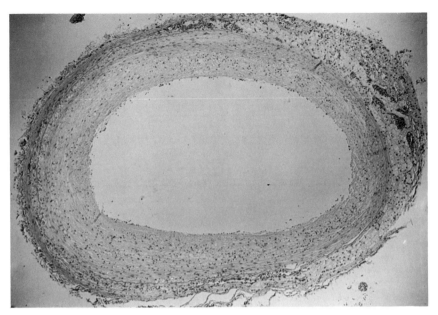

FIG 6–5.
Histologic section of a rabbit iliac artery four weeks after laser thermal angioplasty with a 1.5-mm Laserprobe demonstrating a large lumen with a thin fibrous neointima without significant cellular proliferation (hematoxylin-eosin, × 80).

Laser Equipment

The laser system at Boston University consisted of a 12-W argon laser system (Optilase, model 900, Trimedyne, Inc) coupled to a sterile disposable 300-μm-diameter core fiberoptic fiber with a 2.0-mm Laserprobe at the tip (Fig 6–6). In one case, the 2.0-mm probe could not be passed through a hard, calcified, 12-cm stenosis and a smaller 1.5-mm probe had to be used to cross the lesion (see Fig 6–6). This novel fiberoptic delivery system can be coupled to other argon laser sources, such as the Cooper Lasersonics argon laser generator used in the procedures performed in Sheffield.[20]

Percutaneous Procedure

The majority of the procedures were performed via percutaneous arterial puncture of the ipsilateral femoral artery with the patient under local anesthesia. An 8 to 8.5 F introducer sheath was placed after cannulation of the superficial femoral artery, and 5,000 units of heparin was administered intraarterially. After initial angiography to verify the lesion, a 2.0-mm Laserprobe was inserted into the introduced sheath and advanced under fluoroscopic guidance to the proximal origin of the lesion. Five- or 10-second pulses of 8 to 13 W of argon laser energy were then delivered to the Laserprobe as it was advanced through the lesion with a continuous motion. Care was taken to keep

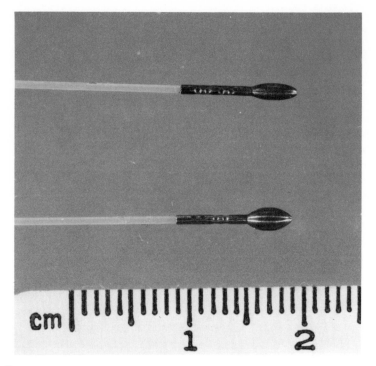

FIG 6–6.
A 1.5-mm Laserprobe *(top)*, and a 2.0-mm Laserprobe *(bottom)*. (From Sanborn TA, Greenfield AJ, Guben JK, et al: Human percutaneous and intraoperative laser thermal angioplasty—Initial clinical results as an adjunct to balloon angioplasty. *J Vasc Surg* 1987; 5:83–90. Reproduced by permission.)

the tip moving as it cooled down after pulse delivery to avoid adherence to the lesion. If adherence was noted on gentle withdrawal of the probe, a repeated laser pulse was delivered to free the probe from the lesion, and a continuous motion was applied to the tip during the subsequent cooling period. Progress of the probe through the lesion was monitored fluoroscopically with several injections of 3 to 5 ml of contrast solution given through the arterial sheath to confirm the position of the Laserprobe. After the lesions were crossed with the Laserprobe, one final pulse was delivered on slow withdrawal of the probe through the lesion to maximize the luminal diameter. The Laserprobe was then removed and an angiogram performed to verify the luminal diameter produced by the procedure.

As the luminal diameter produced by laser thermal angioplasty with the current 2.0-mm diameter Laserprobe was considered inadequate in these large peripheral vessels, the laser procedure was followed in all cases by conventional balloon angioplasty to obtain a definitive lumen, which was verified by a final angiogram. The arterial sheath was subsequently removed and heparin was administered for 24 hours unless a hematoma was present. The patients were discharged within 48 to 72 hours receiving 75 to 325 mg of aspirin a day.

Luminal diameters before, after the Laserprobe, and after the balloon angioplasty were measured by calipers at the narrowest point on the angiograms using a correction for magnification.

Intraoperative Procedure

In two patients at Boston University, either marked obesity or high-grade proximal superficial femoral artery disease precluded a safe percutaneous approach. In these cases, with the patients under local anesthesia and mild sedation, a small cutdown was made to expose the common femoral artery for direct arterial puncture and subsequent laser and balloon angioplasty through an 8.5 F sheath.

Initial Clinical Results

At Boston University, the results of this laser-assisted balloon angioplasty procedure have been classified as follows.

Angiographic and Clinical Success.—This was defined as an improvement in the angiographic luminal diameter, relief of symptoms, improved pulse, or an increase in the Doppler ankle-brachial index by greater than 0.10.

Angiographic Success but Immediate Clinical Failure.—In this group, some improvement in the angiographic luminal diameter was observed; however, the angiographic appearance was less than ideal (small luminal diameters, significant luminal irregularities). Symptoms were not relieved, and the Doppler index did not increase.

Recurrence.—Return of symptoms after an initial clinical success was considered a recurrence and was confirmed by repeated angiography.

In our initial clinical series at Boston University, laser thermal angioplasty with the Laserprobe successfully recanalized six of seven occlusions and partially enlarged the luminal diameters of eight stenoses for a 93% (14/15) angiographic success rate.[21] One to 15 laser pulses were required to traverse the lesions with the Laserprobe; a greater number of pulses were required for longer or more calcified lesions. The angiographic and noninvasive results for this initial group of 15 vessels are summarized in Table 6–2.

One tortuous, calcified, superficial femoral artery occlusion, 4 cm long, was recanalized approximately 2 to 3 cm before tortuosity precluded what was considered further safe advancement. Therefore, the Laserprobe was withdrawn and the remaining 1 to 2 cm was successfully recanalized by a guide wire and subsequent balloon dilation. For the combined procedure, angiographic and clinical success was obtained in 12 (80%) of 15 vessels, with inadequate balloon dilation being the limiting factor in three patients. In the 12 successful procedures, laser recanalization markedly facilitated the negotiation of the lesion by the guide wire and eased the advancement of the balloon catheter through the lesion such that forceful passage was diminished. Repre-

TABLE 6–2.
Angiographic and Noninvasive Results of Thermal Laser Angioplasty Plus Balloon Dilation in the First 15 Procedures*†

VESSEL	LESION	LENGTH, CM	LUMINAL DIAMETER, MM			ANKLE-BRACHIAL DOPPLER INDEX		FOLLOW-UP, MO
			PRELASER	POSTLASER	POSTBALLOON	BEFORE	24–72 HR	
			Angiographic and Clinical Success					
SFA	O	1	0.0	2.0	3.0	0.61	0.81	9
SFA	S	6	0.7	1.5	3.0	0.34	0.69	8
SFA	O	1	0.0	1.8	3.2	0.42	0.94	8
Popliteal	S	1	1.0	1.8	3.2	0.37	0.67	8
SFA	O, S	1, 16	0.0	2.0	4.5	0.38	0.99	7
SFA	S	1	1.1	2.0	4.5	0.49	0.80	7
SFA	S	1	1.7	2.2	4.5	0.50	0.79	6
Popliteal	O	6	0.0	2.0	3.0	0.50	0.79	6
SFA	S	14	0.8	2.0	3.0	0.57	0.78	6
SFA	S	12	0.8	1.5	4.5	0.53	0.69	5
SFA	S	4	0.5	1.5	3.0	0.32	0.42	3
SFA	O	4	0.0	0.0	3.0	0.35	0.53	1
Mean ± SD	. . .	6 ± 5	0.6 ± 0.5	1.7 ± 0.6	3.5 ± 0.7	0.45 ± .09	0.74 ± 0.15	6
			Angiographic Success, Clinical Failure					
SFA	S	39	1.8	2.6	2.6	0.29	0.29	8
SFA	O	26	0.0	1.4	1.4	0.43	0.43	8
SFA	O	6	0.0	1.8	1.9	0.27	0.27	4
Mean ± ISD	. . .	24 ± 14	0.6 ± 0.8	1.9 ± 0.5	2.0 ± 0.5	0.33 ± 0.07	0.33 ± 0.07	6

*From Sanborn TA, Greenfield AJ, Guben JK, et al: Human percutaneous and intraoperative laser thermal angioplasty—Initial clinical results as an adjunct to balloon angioplasty. *J Vasc Surg* 1987; 5:83–90. Reproduced by permission.
†SFA indicates superficial femoral artery; O, occlusion; S, stenosis.

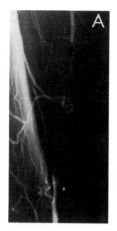 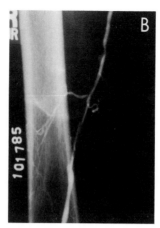 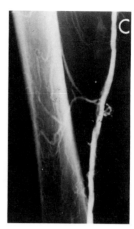

FIG 6–7.
Angiograms of a 6-cm high-grade stenosis of the superficial femoral artery **(A)** in which the luminal diameter was enlarged with the Laserprobe **(B)**. This allowed conventional balloon angioplasty to be performed more easily **(C)**. (From Sanborn TA, Greenfield AJ, Guben JK, et al: Human percutaneous and intraoperative laser thermal angioplasty—Initial clinical results as an adjunct to balloon angioplasty. *J Vasc Surg* 1987; 5:83–90. Reproduced by permission.)

sentative angiographic examples of successful procedures are shown in Figures 6–7 and 6–8.

Three patients with 6-, 26-, and 39-cm hard, calcified lesions were recanalized with the Laserprobe; however, balloon angioplasty failed to further enlarge the lumen on angiography (see Table 6–2). Clinical evaluation for relief of symptoms or an increase in Doppler index also indicated an inadequate result. All three of these patients underwent elective femoropopliteal bypass

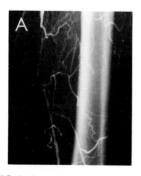 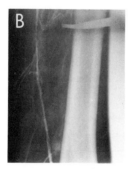 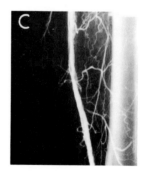

FIG 6–8.
Angiograms of a 4-cm total occlusion of the superficial femoral artery **(A),** which was recanalized with three pulses of 12 W of argon laser energy delivered to the Laserprobe for 10 seconds' duration each **(B)**. This was followed by balloon angioplasty to yield a good angiographic result **(C)**. (From Sanborn TA, Greenfield AJ, Guben JK, et al: Human percutaneous and intraoperative laser thermal angioplasty—Initial clinical results as an adjunct to balloon angioplasty. *J Vasc Surg* 1987; 5:83–90. Reproduced by permission.)

surgery. Of note, two of these patients with long lesions (26 and 39 cm) were also bypass failures, indicating the diffuse nature of the disease.

No major complications were encountered in this investigational study (i.e., perforation, emergency surgery, distal embolization, or limb loss). Minor complications included a small groin hematoma in three patients, minimal thrombus adherent to the tip of the Laserprobe in six patients, and one detachment of the metallic tip during the procedure. This detachment of the Laserprobe tip was easily recognized fluoroscopically, and an attached 0.016-in. safety wire allowed for prompt removal without complications. Further tip detachment has been avoided with new Laserprobe design modifications.

All patients had follow-up examinations at 1, 3, and 6 months, when possible. Of the 12 procedures with initial angiographic and clinical success, asymptomatic status and good Doppler indexes (0.73 ± 0.21) were present in ten cases (83%) during the initial follow-up period of 1 to 9 months (mean, 6 months). Two patients had recurrence of symptoms and underwent repeated angiography. One patient (see Table 6–2, patient 2), a diabetic with rest pain and poor distal runoff, had recurrence of symptoms 2 months after the procedure. Angiography revealed not only occlusion of the superficial femoral artery but significant progression of an abdominal aortic stenosis, which required axillofemoral bypass. The second patient (see Table 6–2, patient 5), a diabetic and heavy smoker with rest pain and poor distal runoff, developed recurrence of symptoms 4 months after the procedure. Repeated angiography demonstrated a patent laser segment, a 1-cm occlusion that had been recanalized, but restenosis of a 16-cm-length balloon-dilated stenotic segment.

In this initial FDA-approved clinical series, laser thermal angioplasty with the Laserprobe, served as a useful adjunct to conventional peripheral balloon angioplasty with 100% safety and a 93% (14/15) angiographic recanalization rate. For the combined laser and balloon procedure, the initial clinical success rate was 80%, or 12 of 15 vessels. Two of the clinical failures were in diabetic patients with long lesions (26 and 39 cm) and poor distal runoff who also had bypass failure. These results represent a significant advancement over previously published clinical trials of percutaneous laser angioplasty in peripheral vessels using bare fiberoptic fibers. Reporting on their clinical experience in 16 patients using argon laser radiation through a bare fiberoptic fiber, Ginsberg et al.[15] observed an improved angiographic lumen in only 47% (8/17) of vessels attempted, whereas vessel perforation occurred in three patients, spasm in four patients, and severe heat-related pain in seven patients. These initial results of Laserprobe recanalization plus balloon dilation also compare favorably with published 2-year patency rates of 56% to 84% for femoropopliteal balloon angioplasty.[24]

The improvement in safety and efficacy of laser recanalization of peripheral vessels in the present study is attributed to the Laserprobe design, in which argon laser energy is used to heat a rounded metallic tip. Histologic studies in atherosclerotic rabbit iliac arteries indicate that one aspect of the safety of the Laserprobe lies in the evenly distributed circumferential removal of the atherosclerotic lesion by laser thermal energy.[11] The rounded tip also assisted in maintaining a coaxial position to prevent vessel perforation.

The small, recanalized channel of 1.7 mm created by the 2-mm Laserprobe precluded sole use of the laser device to disobliterate these large peripheral vessels, and balloon angioplasty was required to obtain an adequate angiographic luminal diameter. Since fracture and dissection of the arterial wall after balloon angioplasty may lead to restenosis, ideally one may want to remove the obstructing lesion as completely as possible and to leave behind a smooth, nonthrombogenic residual arterial surface. An appropriately sized Laserprobe for the vessel to be treated may accomplish this goal. Thus, the present 1.5- and 2.0-mm Laserprobes may be ideal for distal tibial or possibly coronary vessels, and larger Laserprobes may be required for the larger peripheral vessels. These larger sizes may preclude a percutaneous approach necessitating an open intraoperative technique.

Use of the Laserprobe to Recanalize Total Arterial Occlusions

A recent report of the combined experience at Northern General Hospital and Boston University Medical Center was directed toward the use of the Laserprobe to increase the initial success rate in the recanalization of totally occluded peripheral arteries.[20] In this series, 50 (89%) of 56 femoropopliteal occlusions were successfully traversed by the Laserprobe to provide an initial channel for subsequent balloon dilation. The Laserprobe crossed all 17 occlusions that were subjectively classified as easy to recanalize by conventional means, and 19 of 21 lesions considered difficult to cross by standard balloon angioplasty. The Laserprobe was also successful in 14 of 18 occlusions judged impossible to treat by conventional angioplasty. Since there were two acute reocclusions, the overall initial clinical success rate was 86%. This compares quite favorably with recent large series of conventional balloon angioplasty.[25, 26] One European series reported an overall success rate of 72% in 286 femoropopliteal occlusions,[25] whereas a more recent series from Johns Hopkins Hospital, Baltimore, reported an 84% technical success rate and a 78% clinical success rate in 59 femoropopliteal occlusions.[26] Although case selection may vary somewhat in different series, for an initial clinical study using a prototype laser device, the present Laserprobe series compares quite favorably with these other series using conventional balloon angioplasty.

FUTURE DIRECTIONS

Laser thermal angioplasty with an argon laser–heated Laserprobe has been found to have improved safety and efficacy compared with prior clinical studies with bare fiberoptic fibers.[15, 16] The next step will be to determine the exact clinical role of laser thermal angioplasty with a laser probe. Potential clinical applications include the following:

1. To increase the initial success rate in total occlusions or lesions that are difficult to cross and dilate by conventional guidewires and balloon catheters.
2. To decrease the recurrence rate by removing (vaporizing) the lesion rather than merely stretching and "cracking" the lesions.[27]
3. To develop a surgical cutdown approach for larger laser probes to create larger channels in peripheral vessels so that balloon angioplasty is not required.
4. To consider earlier intervention for claudication if the safety of the procedure is verified.
5. To ultimately develop a coronary application.

Preliminary follow-up results in our first 124 femoropopliteal lesions treated with the Laserprobe revealed an overall 72%, 1-year clinical patency (Sanborn TA, et al., unpublished data). Interestingly, however, in short occlusions (1 to 3 cm) and in all stenotic lesions, the 1-year clinical patency is 90% to 95%. If this result is reproducible, it would indicate that laser thermal angioplasty could play a useful role in decreasing recurrence after balloon angioplasty.

Meanwhile, initial clinical trials are also underway to test the feasibility of percutaneous coronary laser thermal angioplasty.[28, 29] While the results are encouraging, it is still too early to make conclusions.

In summary, the use of flexible fiberoptic fibers to transmit laser energy for the ablation of atherosclerotic obstructions does have significant potential in the cardiovascular area, and initial clinical trials indicate that some of the early limitations of laser angioplasty can be solved. What remains to be determined is the exact clinical role of this emerging technology in relation to the current, accepted procedures of bypass surgery and balloon angioplasty.

REFERENCES

1. Gruentzig A: Results of coronary angioplasty and implications for the future. *Am Heart J* 1982; 103:779–783.
2. Meier B, King SB, Gruentzig AR, et al: Repeat coronary angioplasty. *J Am Coll Cardiol* 1984; 4:463–466.
3. Levine S, Ewels CJ, Rosing DR, et al: Coronary angioplasty—Clinical and angiographic follow-up. *Am J Cardiol* 1985; 55:673–676.
4. Holmes DR, Vlietstra RE, Reeder GS, et al: Angioplasty in total coronary occlusions. *J Am Coll Cardiol* 1984; 3:845–849.
5. Kereiakes DJ, Selman MR, McAuley BJ, et al: Angioplasty in total coronary artery occlusion—Experience pressure in 76 consecutive patients. *J Am Coll Cardiol* 1985; 6:526–533.
6. Marcruz R, Martins JRM, Turpinanba AS, et al: Therapeutic possibilities of laser beams in atheromas. *Arq Bras Cardiol* 1980; 34:9–12.

7. Lee G, Ikeda RM, Kozina J, et al: Laser dissolution of coronary atherosclerotic obstruction. *Am Heart J* 1981; 102:1074.

8. Abela GS, Normann S, Cohen D, et al: Effects of carbon dioxide Nd-YAG and argon laser radiation on coronary atheromatous plaque. *Am J Cardiol* 1982; 50:1199–1205.

9. Choy DSJ, Stertzer S, Rotterdam HZ, et al: Transluminal laser catheter angioplasty. *Am J Cardiol* 1982; 50:1006–1008.

10. Choy DSJ, Stertzer SH, Rotterdam HZ, et al: Laser coronary angioplasty—Experience with nine cadaver hearts. *Am J Cardiol* 1982; 50:1209–1211.

11. Sanborn TA, Faxon DP, Haudenschild C, et al: Experimental angioplasty—Circumferential distribution of laser thermal energy with a laser probe. *J Am Coll Cardiol* 1985; 5:934–938.

12. Abela GS, Normann SJ, Cohen DM, et al: Laser recanalization of occluded atherosclerotic arteries in vivo and in vitro. *Circulation* 1985; 71:403–411.

13. Abela GS, Fenech A, Crea F, et al: Hot-tip—Another method of laser vascular recanalization. *Lasers Surg Med* 1985; 5:327–335.

14. Ginsberg R, Kim DS, Guthaner D, et al: Salvage of an ischemic limb by laser angioplasty—Description of a new technique. *Clin Cardiol* 1984; 7:54–58.

15. Ginsberg R, Wexler L, Mitchell RS, et al: Percutaneous transluminal laser angioplasty for treatment of peripheral vascular disease: Clinical experience with 16 patients. *Radiology* 1985; 156:619–624.

16. Choy DSJ, Stertzer SH, Myler RK, et al: Human coronary laser recanalization. *Clin Cardiol* 1984; 7:377–381.

17. Geschwind H, Boussignac G, Teissiere B, et al: Percutaneous transluminal laser angioplasty in man. *Lancet* 1984; 1:844.

18. Livesay JJ, Leachman DR, Hagan PJ, et al: Preliminary report of laser coronary endarterectomy in patients, abstracted. *Circulation* 1985; 72:(Suppl 3)302.

19. Sanborn TA, Cumberland DC, Taylor DI, et al: Human percutaneous laser thermal angioplasty, abstracted. *Circulation* 1985; 72:(Suppl 3)303.

20. Cumberland DC, Sanborn TA, Taylor DI, et al: Percutaneous laser thermal angioplasty—Initial clinical results with a laserprobe in total peripheral artery occlusions. *Lancet* 1986; 1:1457–1459.

21. Sanborn TA, Greenfield AJ, Guben JK, et al: Human percutaneous and intraoperative laser thermal angioplasty—Initial clinical results as an adjunct to balloon angioplasty. *J Vasc Surg* 1987; 5:83–90.

22. Abela GS, Seeger JM, Barbieri E, et al: Laser angioplasty with angioscopic guidance in humans. *J Am Coll Cardiol* 1986; 8:184–192.

23. Sanborn TA, Haudenschild CC, Faxon DP, et al: Angiographic and histologic follow-up of laser angioplasty with a laser probe, abstracted. *J Am Coll Cardiol* 1985; 5:408.

24. Krepel VM, van Andel GJ, van Erp WFM, et al: Percutaneous transluminal angioplasty of the femoropopliteal artery—Initial and long term results. *Radiology* 1985; 156:325–328.

25. Zeitler E, Richter EI, Seyferth W: Femoropopliteal arteries, in Dotter CT, Gruentzig A, Schoop W, et al (eds): *Percutaneous Transluminal Angioplasty.* New York, Springer-Verlag New York, 1983, pp 105–127.

26. Hewes RC, White RI, Murray RR, et al: Long-term results of superficial femoral artery angioplasty. *Am J Radiol* 1986; 146:1025–1032.

27. Sanborn TA, Faxon DP, Haudenschild CC, et al: The mechanism of transluminal angioplasty—Evidence for formation of aneurysms in experimental atherosclerosis. *Circulation* 1983; 68:1136–1140.
28. Cumberland DC, Starkey IR, Oakley GDG: Percutaneous laser-assisted coronary angioplasty. *Lancet* 1986; 1:214.
29. Sanborn TA, Faxon DP, Kellett MA, et al: Percutaneous coronary laser thermal angioplasty. *J Am Coll Cardiol* 1986; 8:1437–1440.

7

Laser Endarterectomy

John Eugene, M.D.

Endarterectomy is a fundamental technique of reconstructive cardiovascular surgery and is usually performed to remove an obstructing or ulcerating atheroma from an artery.[1-3] The diseased intima and underlying internal elastic lamina are dissected away from the wall of the artery to leave a luminal surface lined by the innermost fibers of the media. Since the introduction of endarterectomy 40 years ago, it has become evident that removing the intima of a diseased artery enables one to restore normal blood flow and achieve long-term patency of the artery.[4] This chapter describes work that we have performed at the University of California at Irvine evaluating the treatment of experimental atherosclerosis using laser endarterectomy.[5-9]

TECHNIQUE OF LASER ENDARTERECTOMY

To perform a laser endarterectomy, we dissect the artery free of surrounding tissues. Following systemic anticoagulation with heparin, proximal and distal vascular control of the artery is obtained and a longitudinal opening is made in the artery to visualize the atheroma. A line of laser craters is created at the proximal and the distal ends of an atheroma using individual laser exposures. The lines of laser craters are connected by continuous laser radiation to form the sites for future proximal and distal end points. This maneuver loosens the atheroma from the artery just beneath the internal elastic lamina and exposes the cleavage plane. The plaque is dissected free from the artery by gently retracting the plaque and using constant laser light to dissect within the cleavage plane and free the plaque from the artery. Once the plaque is removed, any remaining particles of atheromatous debris can be vaporized by individual laser exposures, and the end points can be fused (welded) for a smooth and secure transition from endarterectomy surface to intima. This technique is illustrated in Figure 7–1 and Plates 8 and 9.

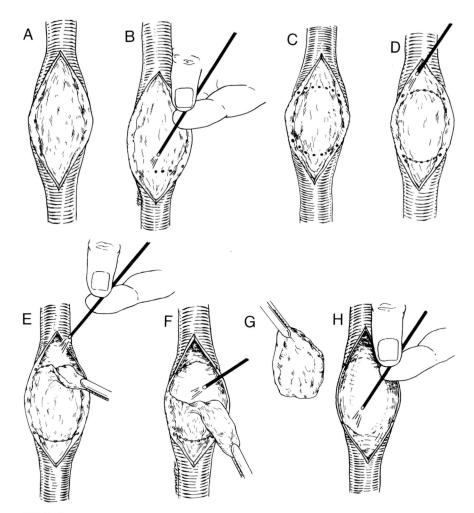

FIG 7–1.
A, artist's drawing of an arteriosclerotic artery opened longitudinally to expose an atheroma.
B, lines of laser craters are being created at one end of the atheroma by individual laser exposures. **C,** individual laser exposures have been applied to create lines of laser craters at both ends of the atheroma. **D,** the lines of laser craters are connected by continuous laser radiation to loosen the atheroma and create the sites for the proximal and distal end points. **E,** the atheroma is being elevated away from the artery by continuous applications of laser light. **F,** continuous laser exposures are used to develop the cleavage plane within the media and dissect the atheroma from the artery. **G,** the dissection is completed and the atheroma is removed from the artery. **H,** the proximal and distal end points are welded by continuous laser radiation. (From Eugene JA, McColgan SJ, Hammer-Wilson M, et al: Laser endarterectomy. *Lasers Surg Med* 1985; 5:265–274. Reproduced by permission.)

Our laser endarterectomy technique was developed using the rabbit arteriosclerosis model and the argon ion laser.[5,6] Arteriosclerosis was created in adult New Zealand white rabbits by inflicting balloon catheter trauma to the thoracoabdominal aorta with the rabbits under general anesthesia (intramuscular acepromazine, 0.5 mg/kg; xylazine, 3.0 mg/kg; ketamine, 50 mg/kg) and maintaining them on a 2% cholesterol diet for 20 weeks. Early in our experience, we performed angiography on the rabbits to evaluate the severity of arteriosclerosis and we learned that significant arteriosclerotic lesions were produced in 86% of surviving rabbits. Grossly, the diseased aortas are thickened and discolored (white with yellow streaks), and the disease is uniform throughout the traumatized aorta. Microscopically, each atheroma has a fibrous cap that overlies areas of fatty infiltration (foam cells), inflammation, and focal calcifications with fracture of the internal elastic lamina and extension into the superficial fibers of the media.

LASER ENDARTERECTOMY VS. CONVENTIONAL ENDARTERECTOMY

Although we had demonstrated that laser energy could be used to perform an endarterectomy, there was no proof that it was different from standard endarterectomy. A series of experiments was performed to compare endarterectomy by laser and endarterectomy by knife.[7] A thoracoabdominal exploration was performed in 16 arteriosclerotic rabbits under general anesthesia. The aorta was isolated, and heparin (3.0 mg/kg intravenously) was administered. Proximal and distal vascular control was obtained, and the aorta was opened longitudinally. In eight rabbits, open laser endarterectomy was performed with an argon ion laser (Coherent INNOVA 20) with mixed wavelengths of 488 and 514.5 nm transmitted through a 400-μm quartz fiberoptic at a power of 1.0 W. In the remaining eight rabbits, standard surgical endarterectomy was performed.

On completion of the endarterectomy, the aortas were removed, preserved, serially sectioned at 6-μm intervals, and stained with hematoxylin-eosin for histologic examination. The specimens were assigned a point score determined by the gross and microscopic surface characteristics (1, arterial perforation; 2, the wrong cleavage plane; 3, rough surface; 4, smooth surface) and by the type of transition at the endarterectomy end points (1, arterial perforation; 2, intimal flap; 3, rough transition; and 4, smooth transition).

By gross appearance, satisfactory endarterectomy surfaces were obtained with both techniques. The end points following laser endarterectomy appeared to be more even and more well defined than the end points following conventional endarterectomy. By microscopic appearance, both techniques showed that the endarterectomy surfaces were in the proper cleavage plane, with removal of the diseased intima and internal elastic laminae, and were relatively smooth and free of debris (Figs 7–2 and 7–3). The end points, however, were

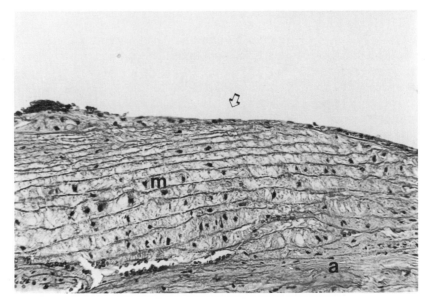

FIG 7–2.
Longitudinal section of an arteriosclerotic rabbit aorta following conventional endarterectomy showing that the atheroma and internal elastic lamina have been removed. The endarterectomy surface *(open arrow)* is smooth and the elastic fibers of the media *(m)* retain their normal configuration; *a* indicates adventitia (hematoxylin-eosin, × 40).

quite different. The conventional endarterectomy end points exhibited a rough transition from media to intima (Fig 7–4), and in two cases, intimal flaps were seen (Fig 7–5). The laser endarterectomy end points were welded in place. Most of the laser end points exhibited a smooth transition from media to intima, and there were no distal intimal flaps (Fig 7–6). When the surfaces were graded, both conventional and laser endarterectomy specimens achieved identical scores of 3.6. When the end points were graded, the conventional endarterectomy specimens achieved a score of 2.8 and the laser endarterectomy score was 3.6 ($P < 0.05$). These experiments demonstrated that laser endarterectomy offers the distinct advantage of welding the end points for a secure transition from endarterectomy surface to arterial lumen.

EXPERIMENTAL ENDARTERECTOMY COMPARING LASERS

The standard surgical lasers that have been evaluated most extensively for experimental treatment of atherosclerosis include the neodymium:yttrium-aluminum-garnet (Nd:YAG) (1.06 μm), carbon dioxide (10.6 μm), and argon ion laser.[10–12] The technique of laser endarterectomy was developed with the argon ion laser because its beam is within the visible spectrum (488 and 514.5 nm), permitting the surgeon accurately to direct the beam to the target tissue and observe if there is any scatter or transmission of laser light. Additional

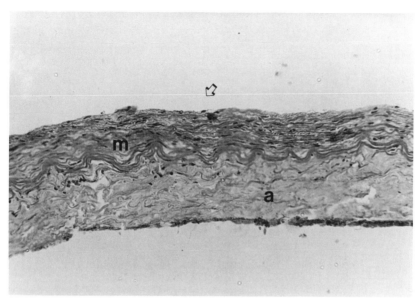

FIG 7–3.
Longitudinal section of an arteriosclerotic rabbit aorta following argon ion laser endarterectomy showing smooth endarterectomy surface *(open arrow)*. The atheroma and the internal elastic lamina have been removed, leaving the elastic fibers of the media *(m)* undisturbed; *a* indicates adventitia (hematoxylin-eosin, × 40).

studies were performed to compare the laser-atheroma interaction of all three lasers by their ability to perform open laser endarterectomy in arteriosclerotic rabbit aortas.[7–9]

The argon ion laser (Coherent INNOVA 20) beam was delivered through a 400-μm quartz fiberoptic at a power of 1.0 W. The Nd:YAG laser (Molectron Medical Model 8000-3) beam was delivered through a 600-μm quartz fiberoptic with integral aiming light at a power of 10 to 20 W. Carbon dioxide laser (Directed Energy model systems LS 20-H) energy was delivered directly from the laser head to the aorta at a power of 10 W for 10 msec (0.01 J). Laser endarterectomy was performed in arteriosclerotic rabbits with each of the lasers, and the aortas were resected for histologic study following the procedures.

Grossly, the argon ion laser endarterectomies appeared satisfactory. The surfaces were smooth, without residual atheroma, and the end points were welded in place. Grossly, the Nd:YAG laser endarterectomies appeared unsatisfactory. The surfaces were dessicated and the end points were burned. Significant thermal injury was seen in the adventitia of the aortas and in surrounding structures, such as the inferior vena cava, indicating transmission of Nd:YAG energy through the arteriosclerotic aortas. The carbon dioxide laser endarterectomies appeared generally satisfactory by gross inspection; however, closer inspection under a dissecting microscope revealed that fragments of

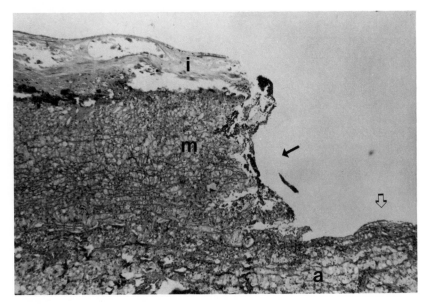

FIG 7–4.
Longitudinal section of a distal end point following conventional endarterectomy in an arterio-sclerotic rabbit aorta showing an abrupt transition from endarterectomy surface *(open arrow)* to atheroma *(closed arrow); i* indicates intima; *m,* media; *a,* adventitia (hematoxylin-eosin, × 10).

intima and internal elastic lamina were left on the surfaces, and there were minute perforations at the end points.

Microscopically, the argon ion laser endarterectomy surfaces showed the cleavage plane to be just beneath the internal elastic lamina in all of the experiments. The surfaces all appeared relatively smooth. The end points were welded securely for an even transition from media to intima. The Nd:YAG laser endarterectomy surfaces showed thermal changes manifested as charring and discoloration. The depth of the cleavage plane was irregular and was seen to be superficial to the media or too deep within the media (Fig 7–7). Perforation occurred at the distal end points in 75% of the experiments (Fig 7–8). Despite the fact that the gross appearance of the carbon dioxide laser endarterectomy surfaces and end points was satisfactory, microscopically the surfaces were uneven and were often in the wrong cleavage plane (Fig 7–9). Perforations occurred at the distal end points in 80% of the carbon dioxide endarterectomies (Fig 7–10).

Argon ion laser endarterectomy achieved a surface score of 3.6 and an end point score of 3.5. The Nd:YAG laser endarterectomy achieved a surface score of 2.6 and an end point score of 1.5. Carbon dioxide laser endarterectomy achieved a surface score of 2.3 and an end point score of 1.3. Argon ion laser endarterectomy required an average energy density of 110 ± 12 J/sq cm. The Nd:YAG laser endarterectomy required an average energy density of 1147 ±

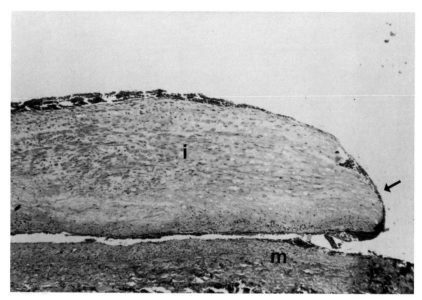

FIG 7–5.
Longitudinal section of a distal end point following conventional endarterectomy in an arteriosclerotic rabbit aorta showing separation of the layers of the arterial wall at the transition from media *(m)* to intima *(i) (closed arrow)*. This represents a distal intimal flap (hematoxylin-eosin, × 10).

120 J/sq cm, and carbon dioxide laser endarterectomy required a mean energy density of 38 ± 5 J/sq cm.

These data showed that argon ion and carbon dioxide laser radiation were well absorbed by atheromas, but Nd:YAG laser radiation was not well absorbed and was transmitted and scattered to surrounding tissues. The excellent interaction between atheromas and carbon dioxide laser energy did not result in a satisfactory endarterectomy because the beam could not be accurately delivered without fiberoptics. The poor laser-atheroma interaction observed with the Nd:YAG laser led to an unsatisfactory endarterectomy even though fiberoptic delivery was available. Satisfactory endarterectomy was performed only with the argon ion laser because the energy was well absorbed by arteriosclerotic rabbit aortas and the beam was accurately directed through a fiberoptic.

PHOTOSENSITIZATION OF ATHEROMAS

Neoplasms are known to accumulate hematoporphyrin derivative (HPD), and this accumulation of HPD can be detected by fluorescence of the tumor under ultraviolet light. When neoplasms are photosensitized with HPD, exposure to specific wavelengths of laser light causes a cytotoxic reaction that destroys the tumor. Theoretically, if atheromas can be photosensitized in a similar fashion, selective ablation of atheromas could be accomplished with laser

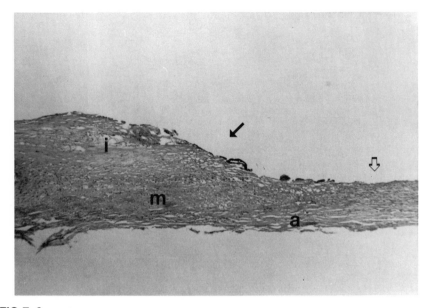

FIG 7–6.
Longitudinal section of a distal end point following argon ion laser endarterectomy in an arteriosclerotic rabbit aorta showing a smooth transition from endarterectomy surface *(open arrow)* to intima *(closed arrow).* The layers of the end point are welded together to prevent an intimal flap; *i* indicates intima; *m,* media; *a,* adventitia (hematoxylin-eosin, × 10).

light using energy levels so low that injury to adjacent tissue would be eliminated and the threat of arterial perforation would be greatly reduced.

Fluorescence of arteriosclerotic arteries that have been treated with HPD has been described in rabbits, a Patas monkey, and human cadaver aortas.[13–16] An additional study was performed to determine the site of localization of porphyrins in arteriosclerotic arteries.[17] Photofrin II was used instead of HPD because it is the current commercial preparation of porphyrin used for photodynamic therapy of cancer. Four groups of rabbits were studied: normal rabbits; normal rabbits given 5 mg/kg of Photofrin II intravenously; arteriosclerotic rabbits; and arteriosclerotic rabbits given 5 mg/kg of Photofrin II intravenously. Within 48 hours the rabbits underwent surgical exploration, and multiple full-thickness biopsies of their aortas were obtained. These biopsies were immediately frozen and sectioned at 4-μm intervals. Adjacent alternate sections were either stained with hematoxylin-eosin or prepared for fluorescence microscopy to quantitate porphyrin fluorescence. Paired sections were matched so that the sites of fluorescence could be localized to a specific histologic region of the arteries. A marked increase in fluorescence was seen in the intima of the arteriosclerotic arteries, proving that porphyrins localized within atheromas (Plate 10).

With the knowledge that porphyrins localized in atheromas, laser endar-

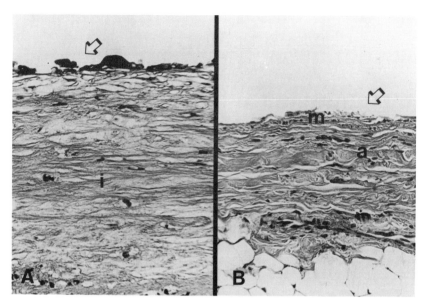

FIG 7–7.
Longitudinal sections of arteriosclerotic rabbit aortas following Nd:YAG laser endarterectomy. **A,** cleavage plane superficial to the media *(m)* with charring of the surface. **B,** cleavage plane deep within the media almost to the adventitia *(a); i* indicates intima (hematoxylin-eosin, × 40).

terectomy was used to determine if the atheromas were photosensitized by the porphyrin accumulation. Laser endarterectomy was performed in arteriosclerotic rabbits given 5 mg/kg of intravenous Photofrin II 48 hours preoperatively, and arteriosclerotic rabbits without Photofrin II pretreatment. An argon ion laser was used because the wavelengths (488 and 514.5 nm) are in the range of one of the best absorption peaks of porphyrins. Laser endarterectomy in arteriosclerotic rabbits required an average energy density of 103 ± 14 J/sq cm, and laser endarterectomy in arteriosclerotic rabbits given Photofrin II required an average density of 33 ± 3 J/sq cm (*P* < .01). Since the technique of laser endarterectomy requires atheromas to be dissected from the artery, the significant changes in energy density show that porphyrin localization in atheromas does indeed sensitize atheromas to selective laser ablation.

FUTURE DIRECTIONS FOR LASER ENDARTERECTOMY

Laser endarterectomy should be evaluated in a long-term animal model to determine healing and long-term patency. In performing these studies, laser endarterectomy should be compared with conventional endarterectomy and laser angioplasty. The arteriosclerotic rabbit preparation is not suitable for

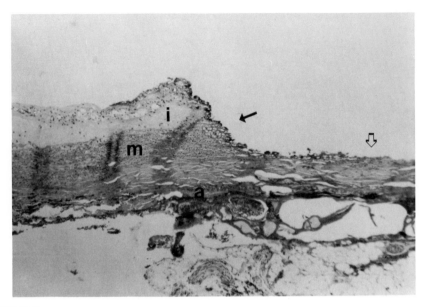

FIG 7–8.
Longitudinal section of a distal end point following Nd:YAG laser endarterectomy in an arteriosclerotic rabbit aorta showing an abrupt transition from endarterectomy surface *(open arrow)* to arterial surface *(closed arrow)*. There is a full-thickness injury (perforation) to the arterial wall at the transition of the end point; *i* indicates intima; *m,* media; *a,* adventitia
(hematoxylin-eosin; × 10).

long-term studies. The most promising animal model for this work appears to
be arteriosclerotic swine.

The thrombogenicity of laser endarterectomy needs to be evaluated. In a
preliminary study, the thrombogenic potential of laser endarterectomy was
found to be identical to the thrombogenicity of conventional endarterectomy.[18]
In this study, the thrombogenicity of laser endarterectomy and conventional
endarterectomy was significantly less than the thrombogenicity of the luminal
surface of a laser angioplasty.

All of the laser endarterectomy studies that have been reported have been
performed with continuous-wave lasers. Preliminary data from our laboratory
using a pulsed laser (frequency doubled Nd:YAG laser, 532 nm, Laserscope)
showed perforations at the end points related to the high peak power of this
laser. Obviously, further work is required evaluating the use of pulsed lasers
for endarterectomy. Laser endarterectomy can also be performed using laser
scalpels made of metal (similar to the "hot-tip") or sapphire crystals. The use
of laser scalpels to perform endarterectomy should simplify the technique and
make the procedure much like the standard endarterectomy with a knife.

Finally, clinical studies of laser endarterectomy should commence. These
can begin with modification of standard techniques, such as welding the end

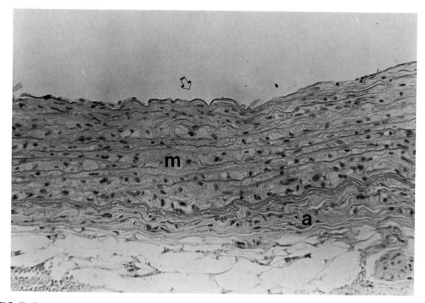

FIG 7–9.
Longitudinal section of an arteriosclerotic rabbit aorta following carbon dioxide laser endarterectomy shows an uneven surface with fragments of the internal elastic lamina left in place (arrow). This endarterectomy surface is in the wrong cleavage plane; *m* indicates media; *a*, adventitia (hematoxylin-eosin, × 40).

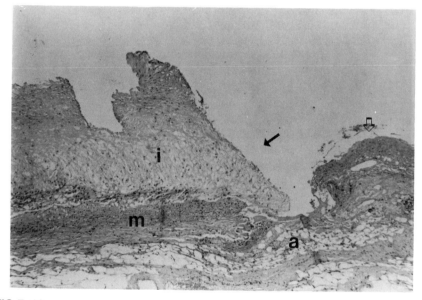

FIG 7–10.
Longitudinal section of a distal end point following carbon dioxide laser endarterectomy in an arteriosclerotic rabbit aorta. The transition from endarterectomy surface *(open arrow)* to arterial surface *(closed arrow)* is uneven and irregular. There is a full-thickness injury (perforation) at the transition of the end point; *i* indicates intima; *m,* media; *a,* adventitia (hematoxylin-eosin, × 40).

points following conventional endarterectomy. As more experience is gained, laser endarterectomy can be used in both the peripheral vascular and coronary artery systems to supplement and perhaps even replace standard bypass procedures.

REFERENCES

1. Wiley EJ, Kerr E, Davies O: Experimental and clinical experiences with use of fascia lata applied as graft about major arteries after thromboendarterectomy and aneurysmography. *Surg Gynecol Obstet* 1951; 93:257–272.
2. Wiley EJ: Thromboendarterectomy for atherosclerotic thrombosis of major arteries. *Surgery* 1952; 32:275–292.
3. Szilagy DE, Smith RF, Whitney DG: The durability of aortoiliac endarterectomy. *Arch Surg* 1964; 89:827–839.
4. Dos Santos JC: From embolectomy to endarterectomy or the fall of a myth. *J Cardiovasc Surg* 1976; 17:113–128.
5. Eugene J, McColgan SJ, Hammer-Wilson M, et al: Laser endarterectomy. *Lasers Surg Med* 1985; 5:265–274.
6. Eugene J, McColgan SJ, Hammer-Wilson M, et al: Laser applications to arteriosclerosis: Angioplasty, angioscopy and open endarterectomy. *Lasers Surg Med* 1985; 5:309–320.
7. Eugene J, McColgan SJ, Pollock ME, et al: Experimental arteriosclerosis treated by conventional and laser endarterectomy. *J Surg Res* 1985; 39:31–38.
8. Eugene J, Pollock ME, McColgan SJ, et al: Fiber optic versus direct laser delivery for endarterectomy of experimental atheromas. *Proc Int Soc Opt Eng* 1985; 576:55–58.
9. Eugene J, McColgan SJ, Pollock ME, et al: Experimental arteriosclerosis treated by argon ion and neodymium-YAG laser endarterectomy. *Circulation* 1985; 72(suppl 2):200–206.
10. Geschwind HJ, Boussignac G, Teisseire B, et al: Conditions for effective Nd:YAG angioplasty. *Br Heart J* 1984; 52:484–498.
11. Livesay JJ, Leachman DR, Hogan PJ, et al: Preliminary report on laser coronary endarterectomy in patients, abstracted. *Circulation* 1985; 72(suppl 3):302.
12. Abela GS, Seeger JM, Barbieri E, et al: Laser angioplasty with angioscopic guidance in humans. *J Am Coll Cardiol* 1986; 8:184–192.
13. Spears JR, Serur J, Shropstire D, et al: Fluorescence of experimental atheromatous plaques with hematoporphyrin derivative. *J Clin Invest* 1983; 71:395–399.
14. Cortis B, Harris DM, Principe J: Angioscopy of hematoporphyrin derivative in experimental atherosclerosis. *Proc Int Cong Appl Lasers Electro-Opt* 1984; 43:128–130.
15. Kessel D, Sykes E: Porphyrin accumulation by atheromatous plaques of the aorta. *Photochem Photobiol* 1984; 40:59–64.
16. Litvak F, Grundfest WS, Forrester JS, et al: Effects of hematoporphyrin derivative and photodynamic therapy on arteriosclerotic rabbits. *Am J Cardiol* 1985; 56:667–671.
17. Pollock ME, Eugene J, Hammer-Wilson M, et al: Photosensitization of experimental atheromas by porphyrins. *J Am Coll Cardiol* 1987; 9:639–646.
18. Pollock ME, Eugene J, Hammer-Wilson M, et al: The thrombogenic potential of argon ion laser endarterectomy. *J Surg Res* 1987; 42:153–158.

8

Laser Vascular Anastomotic Welding*

Rodney A. White, M.D.
George Kopchok, B.S.
Geoffrey H. White, M.D., F.R.A.C.S.
Stanley R. Klein, M.D.
Jouni Uitto, M.D., Ph.D.

Vascular tissue fusion by lasers is performed by directing a low-energy beam at the apposed edges of the repair. The tissues are approximated with stay sutures or nonreflective instruments, and laser energy is passed back and forth over the anastomotic site until fusion is achieved. Vessel welding is apparent to the trained eye, as is nonunion caused by inadequate energy delivery or misaligned edges. Conversely, excessive energy delivery results in obvious tissue coagulation or vaporization. Fiberoptic laser transmission and hand-eye coordination are adequate for repair or anastomosis of vessels with diameters greater than 3 mm, whereas magnification and precise mechanical control of the laser beam are necessary for microanastomoses of smaller vessels. The laser power, and the amount of energy and time required (energy fluence or power density), vary according to the type of laser and the size of the vessels. Although laser repairs can be fashioned in time intervals equal to or slightly longer than those required for suture repairs, the optimum wavelengths and laser parameters for different types of seals are not yet established.

*The experimental work described in this chapter was supported in part by PHS grants HL-32622, GM-28833, AM-28450, and AM-35297 from the National Institutes of Health.

LASER WELDING OF MICROVESSELS

The majority of the published work on the use of lasers to weld vascular anastomoses relates to sealing of micróvessels. Carbon dioxide (CO_2), neodymium:yttrium-aluminum-garnet (Nd:YAG) (1,060 nm), and argon laser welds in microvessels are faster, have no foreign body reaction, and have adequate tensile strength compared with sutured wounds.[1-3] Frazier et al.[4] performed microvascular anastomoses of femoral arteries in growing miniswine and demonstrated that CO_2 laser anastomoses grew normally in diameter whereas sutured controls had restricted growth. McCarthy et al.[5] reported 9% incidence of aneurysms in rabbit carotid artery anastomoses made with the CO_2 laser at 60 to 100 mW power. White et al.[6] noted that optimal fusion, with no aneurysms, occurred at 120 to 130 mW. Epstein and Cooley[7] reported that the optimal CO_2 laser parameters for small-vessel welding were powers of 80 to 120 mW, using 80 to 160 pulses of 0.1-second duration, with spot size of 0.2 mm and 2 to 3 J/sq mm energy fluence. With powers greater than 120 mW, there was increased tissue necrosis and thrombosis.

LASER WELDING OF MEDIUM-SIZED VESSELS

Laser Welding of Veins

Extensive experiments in our laboratory have shown that CO_2, Nd:YAG (1,060 nm), and argon lasers can be used to seal 6- to 8-mm-diameter canine femoral and jugular veins.[8-10] Venotomies 2 cm long were fused using 1 W power over 25 seconds for CO_2, 1 W over 40 seconds for Nd:YAG, and 0.5 W over 240 seconds for the argon laser. All repairs were patent at 1 to 4 weeks without evidence of aneurysms or luminal narrowing. Laser repairs of venotomies were compared with sutured controls and found to have similar healing by biochemical analysis and tensile strength determinations. Histologic examination of the sutured wounds revealed a granulomatous inflammatory reaction around the sutures, with areas of excessive collagen accumulation and disorientation of elastin fiber configuration. In contrast, the laser-welded wounds had minimal inflammatory response, near-normal collagen content, and minimal residual disorientation or breaks in the elastic fiber continuity[9] (Fig 8–1).

Laser Welding of Arteries

Laser welding of medium-sized arteries (>3 mm) presents several unique problems. Thicker walls, pulsatile flow, systemic arterial pressures of 100 to 150 mm Hg, in contrast to the much lower pressures in microvessels and veins, and the inherent contractile properties of arteries produce challenges to weld integrity. In canine studies we have observed that the CO_2 laser energy at 1 to 2 W power (400 to 1,000 J/sq cm fluence) did not produce seals that

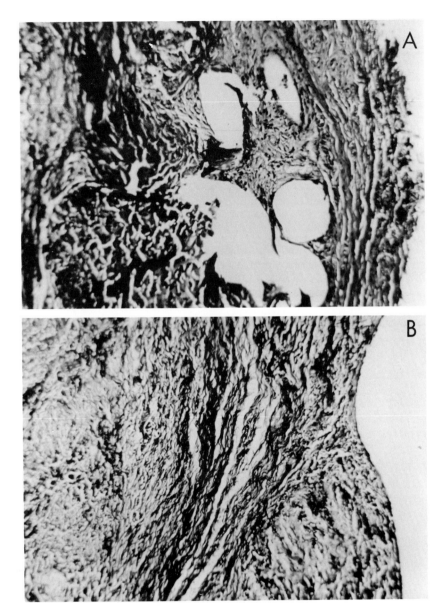

FIG 8–1.
Histologic appearance of sutured and Nd:YAG laser-welded venotomies at 5 weeks. Sutured wounds **(A)** had granulomatous reaction around the sutures, areas of excessive collagen accumulation, and a broad gap in elastin continuity, whereas laser welds **(B)** had near-normal vein architecture (Verhoeff–van Gieson's stain, × 100). (From White RA, Abergel RP, Lyons R, et al: Laser welding—An alternative method of venous repair. *J Surg Res* 1986; 41:260–263. Reproduced by permission.)

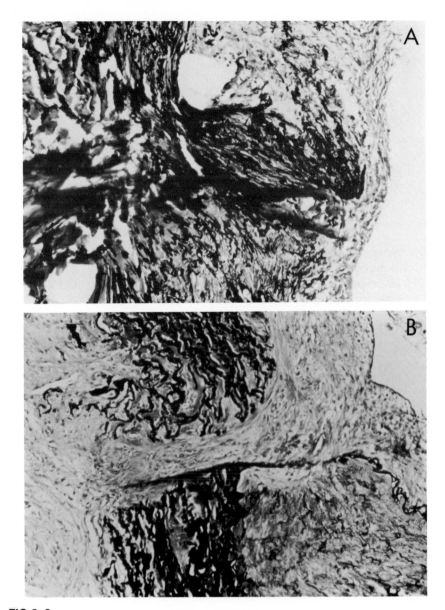

FIG 8–2.
Histologic appearance of sutured **(A)** and argon laser–welded **(B)** arteriotomies at 4 weeks. Sutured wound shows granulomatous reaction around sutures and disorientation of elastin fibers, whereas laser-welded wound has minimal foreign body response and reorienting fibers (Verhoeff–van Gieson's stain, × 100). (From White RA, Kopchok G, Abergel RP, et al: Comparison of laser-welded and sutured arteriotomies. *Arch Surg* 1986; 121:1133–1135. Reproduced by permission.)

could withstand the higher arterial pressure of these larger vessels.[11] The Nd:YAG laser welds in large arteries were initially successful, but the majority failed within 20 to 40 minutes. In contrast, the argon laser sealed 2-cm-long arteriotomies that remained intact and healed within 4 to 6 weeks. Ashworth et al.[12] have recently reported successful end-to-end laser-assisted vascular anastomoses of 4- to 5-mm-diameter canine carotid arteries using a milliwatt CO_2 laser (150 to 175 mW), with successful function for up to 4 weeks.

Additional studies in our laboratory have compared the histologic nature, tensile strength, and collagen synthesis of 2-cm-long argon laser–welded (0.5 W, 240 seconds exposure per 1 cm length of repair) and sutured arteriotomies from 1 to 4 weeks.[13] Laser anastomoses required an average of one suture per repair, whereas 13 sutures per repair were used for sutured arteriotomies. At removal, all experimental closures were patent without hematomas, aneurysms, or luminal dilatation. Histologic examination revealed that laser-welded arteriotomies have less inflammatory reaction, more normal collagen and elastin reorientation, and similar endothelial continuity when compared with the control, sutured wounds (Fig 8–2, Plate 11). The tensile strength of the 1- and 2-week laser specimens was less than that of sutured wounds at 1 and 2 weeks but became approximately equal to that of sutured repairs at 3 and 4 weeks. There were no significant differences in the rates of collagen synthesis.

Laser Welding of Arteriovenous Anastomoses

Based on our preliminary success using the argon laser to seal venotomies and arteriotomies in medium-sized vessels, we have directed our investigations to performing vein-artery anastomoses.[14] Bilateral side-to-side arteriovenous fistulas 2 cm in length were created in dogs by isolating the femoral artery and vein in the upper thigh and anastomosing the walls of adjacent arteriotomy and venotomy incisions. Healing of the repairs was studied at 1, 2, 4, and 8 weeks, with one anastomosis (control) closed with running 6–0 polypropylene sutures and the contralateral anastomosis (experimental) welded with an argon laser. Laser welds were fashioned using 0.5 W power, via a 0.3-mm fiberoptic delivery system held at 1 cm distance from the target spot. The spot size was 0.066 sq cm, with 7.6 W/sq cm power density and 1,830 J/sq cm fluence. Total exposure was 240 seconds using 5-second pulses separated by 0.2-second intervals. Laser-welded arteriovenous fistulas were approximated with a single 6–0 polypropylene suture at each apex of the anastomosis and by traction sutures posteriorly and anteriorly at the midportion of the back and front wall of the repairs (Fig 8–3). The traction sutures were used to appose the edges of the vessels during laser fusion. Thus, laser welding of the ten fistulas was accomplished by sealing 40 segments, each 1 cm long, i.e., four segments per anastomosis. The vessels were continuously cooled by drips of saline solution at room temperature, to prevent thermal damage.[15] Seven of the 40 laser-welded segments required one or two additional interrupted sutures to close small holes that did not fuse adequately.

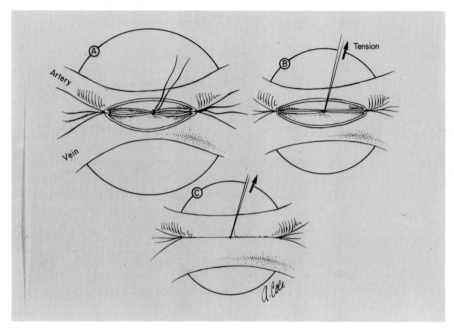

FIG 8–3.
Technique for performing laser welding of vein-artery anastomoses. **A,** sutures are placed at the apices of the incisions and at the middle of the posterior wall; **B,** tension on the suture at the middle of the posterior wall apposes the edges of the repair for welding; **C,** a suture is placed in the middle of the anterior wall and apposes the edges for welding. (From White RA: Technical frontiers for the vascular surgeon: Laser vascular anastomotic welding and angioscopy-assisted intraluminal instrumentation. *J Vasc Surg* 1987; 5:673–680. Reproduced by permission.)

Histologic examination of the seven pairs of control and experimental anastomoses at intervals of 1 to 4 weeks were similar to those described previously for argon laser–welded veins and arteries. At eight weeks, three sets of sutured arteriovenous anastomoses demonstrated intimal hyperplasia at the suture line, whereas no abnormal findings were noted in the laser-welded specimens (Fig 8–4). This observation implicates the sutures in the development of intimal lesions and suggests that laser vein-artery anastomoses may prevent or minimize intimal hyperplastic response. The tensile strengths of both sutured and laser-welded specimens were essentially equivalent from 2 to 8 weeks. The appearance of a canine femoral laser-welded arteriovenous fistula at 16 weeks is shown in Figure 8–5.

Our most recent work has examined vein-artery anastomoses in canine femoral artery bypasses using segments of reversed femoral vein. One anastomosis of the vein bypasses was performed using running 6–0 polypropylene sutures, and the other anastomosis was formed using the same methodology and laser values described for fashioning laser-welded arteriovenous fistulas.

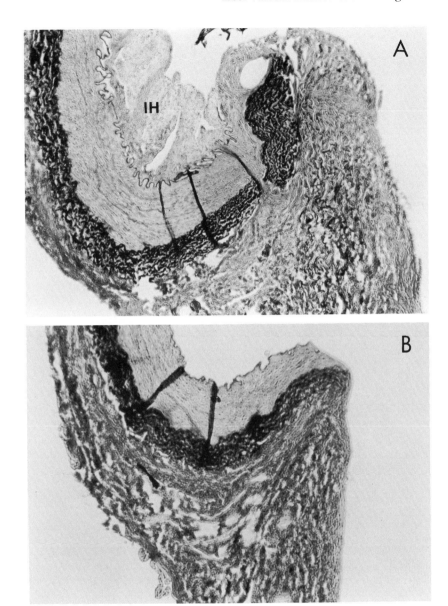

FIG 8–4.
Histologic appearance of 8-week sutured **(A)** and argon laser-welded **(B)** arteriovenous fistulas. The suture's wound has a marked intimal hyperplastic response *(IH)* (Verhoeff–van Gieson's stain, × 40). (From White RA: Technical frontiers for the vascular surgeon: Laser vascular anastomotic welding and angioscopy-assisted intraluminal instrumentation. *J Vasc Surg* 1987; 5:673–680. Reproduced by permission.)

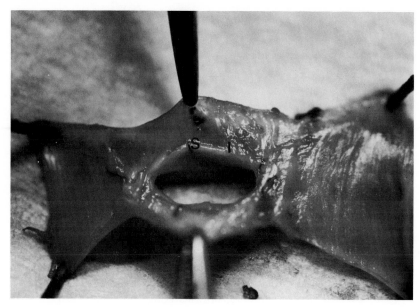

FIG 8–5.
Gross appearance of an argon laser–welded, canine arteriovenous fistula at 16 weeks; *S* indicates traction sutures; *I*, 1-cm lengths of laser fusion.

In these early experiments, laser seals have required only occasional reinforcing sutures, and patency and healing of the bypass grafts has been successful for up to 3 months. This work supports the hypothesis that laser welding of arteriovenous anastomoses is easily performed and may improve long-term patency by eliminating failures related to suture-induced tissue trauma and intimal hyperplasia.

LASER SEALING DURING ENDARTERECTOMY

An additional use for laser vascular sealing has been demonstrated by Eugene et al.[16, 17] Carbon dioxide, Nd:YAG, and argon lasers have been used to perform endarterectomies in an atherosclerotic rabbit model. They have demonstrated that the argon laser can be used to excise isolated segments of atheroma without vessel perforation, and that the intimal end points of the laser dissection became fused to the adjacent arterial wall, forming a smooth transition. In contrast, control of the depth of penetration of the artery was not precise with either CO_2 or Nd:YAG lasers, and each had a significant incidence of vessel perforation. Control endarterectomies performed with a scalpel created intimal flaps at the ends of the incision.

MECHANISM OF LASER VESSEL WELDING

Although the mechanism of vessel sealing by lasers is at present not understood, there appear to be independent effects of laser type and tissue temperature on weld integrity and long-term healing. Serure et al.[2] proposed that tissue adhesion in CO_2 welds of microvascular anastomoses resulted from collagen denaturation in the media and adventitia of the vessel, as well as from fibrin polymerization. Badeau et al.[18] reported that CO_2-assisted microvascular anastomoses are formed in the range of 80 to 120° C. Epstein and Cooley[7] have demonstrated that seals in CO_2 laser–welded microvessels consist of denatured cells and collagen, which reorganize over the first 2 to 4 weeks of healing. They have proposed that a break in the elastin is responsible for the significant incidence of aneurysms (approximately 10%) that form in the early postoperative period. Quigley et al.[19] have shown that the welded areas in CO_2 laser microanastomoses retain a 200- to 300-μm separation of the internal elastic lamina for up to 1 year and that this gap is filled with spindle-shaped cells and has intimal proliferation on the luminal surface.

Intimal hyperplasia is decreased in CO_2 laser–assisted end-to-end microvascular anastomoses of rat femoral arteries compared with sutured controls at 2 weeks but becomes equal by 6 weeks.[20] The authors have postulated that the intimal response at 2 weeks was inhibited by medial injury caused by the CO_2 laser, and that by 6 weeks the vessels had overcome this inhibition. Recent reports of a 5% to 10% incidence of aneurysms in the first month,[5] and intimal thickening at one year,[19] in CO_2-sealed microvessels have associated these phenomena with a break in the elastic lamina at the site of the CO_2 laser fusion. The break in the elastic lamina of the CO_2 repairs is likely due to the tissue necrosis produced by the 80 to 120° C temperatures generated during the fusion.[18] Recently, Ashworth et al.[12] reported successful end-to-end laser-assisted vascular anastomoses of canine carotid arteries using a milliwatt CO_2 laser (150 to 175 mW, 2,400 to 3,550 J/sq cm energy fluence) and noted no aneurysms up to 4 weeks. The investigators attributed the absence of aneurysms in the larger vessels sealed with the milliwatt CO_2 laser compared with the high incidence of aneurysms reported in microvessels to minimal thermal damage of the vessel wall seen in the large-artery repairs.

During preliminary argon laser vascular tissue welding experiments, we observed that the effectiveness of the welding process was improved if the anastomotic site was irrigated with saline solution. Subsequent to that observation, all fusions have been continuously irrigated with saline solution at 3 ml/min. We have recently studied the effect of tissue temperature on the integrity of arteriovenous welds formed with the argon laser.[15, 21] Welds were performed at various power levels, with and without saline irrigation. Temperatures were continuously recorded during the fusions using a thermal camera. One-centimeter welds were performed using powers of 0.50, 0.75, and 1.00 W,

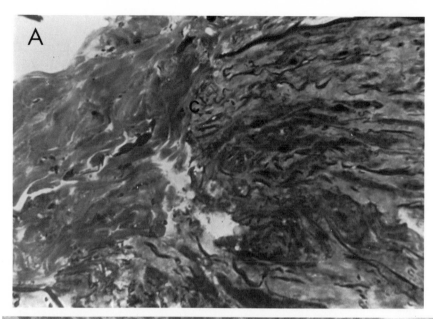

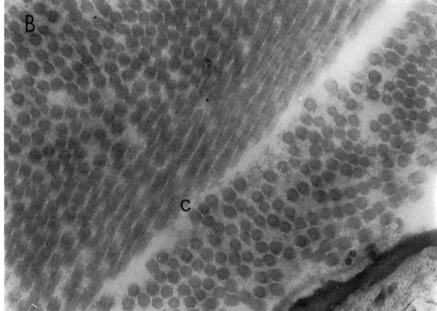

FIG 8–6.
A, histologic examination showing collagen-collagen *(C)* apposition in the media of the vessels (toluidine blue, × 100). **B,** electron micrograph of a collagen-collagen bonding *(C)* (× 27,000). (From White RA, Kopchok G, Peng S: Laser vascular welding—How does it work? *Ann Vasc Surg,* in press. Reproduced by permission.)

with an energy fluence of 1,100 J/sq cm. At 0.50 and 0.75 W, successful welds were formed when the temperatures were 44.2 ± 1.6° C (n = 28) and 55.0 ± 3.6° C (n = 20), with maximum temperatures of 47.9 and 59.9° C, respectively (Plate 12). At 1 W, the tissue was desiccated and the welds were disrupted when exposed to blood flow with temperatures measured at 63.7 ± 10.0° C (n = 22), with a maximum of 88.0° C. Welds were also attempted without saline irrigation at 0.25 and 0.50 W. At 0.25 W, tissue fusion was achieved but disrupted when exposed to intraluminal pressures with temperatures of 50.3 ± 2.0° C (n = 18), and a maximum of 52.6° C. At 0.50 W, the fusion failed after only minimal exposure to the laser energy because of tissue drying, and retraction, with temperatures measured at greater than 125° C (Plate 13). On the basis of these experiments, we concluded that argon laser vascular welding occurs optimally at temperatures between 44 and 60° C, that saline irrigation limits the maximum temperature and prevents drying and retraction of the tissue edges, and that welding at power levels greater than 0.75 W may have deleterious effects.

Histologic and electron microscopic examination of specimens of successful argon laser welds reveal various mechanisms of fusion depending on the alignment and apposition of the vessel edges.[22] Areas that do not have tissue-tissue apposition have a thin layer of coagulated platelets and fibrin forming the interface. Areas of fusion that have direct tissue-tissue apposition demonstrate seals consisting of collagen-collagen bonding in the media of the vessels (Fig 8–6). Apposition between media of vein and intima of artery show that medial collagen and elastin fuse to denatured endothelial cells and the internal elastic membrane of the artery (Fig 8–7). Apposition between media of vein and adventitia of artery show collagen-collagen or collagen-elastin bonding (Fig 8–8). In the areas where the collagen-collagen bonding is apparent, the fusion is evidenced by a prominent blurring and swelling of the collagen ultrastructure (Fig 8–9). The diameters of annealing collagen vary from 100 to 400 μm, whereas unaffected collagen measures less than 70 μm in diameter. Ultrastructurally, annealing collagen appears to be more homogeneous with loss of striations and smearing of the outlines. Elastin also shows somewhat irregular borders.

Our current hypothesis to explain the success of argon laser welding of medium-sized arteries and arteriovenous anastomoses, compared with CO_2 and Nd:YAG failures, is that the CO_2 fusion is formed by a coagulum of denatured collagen and cells produced by temperatures greater than 100° C. This coagulum is adequate to withstand the low pressures found in microvessels and veins but is inadequate to maintain integrity in the presence of higher systemic arterial pressures. The argon laser fusion can be performed in a lower temperature range, which does not denature the collagen and may establish a physiochemical bond by reforming linkages in annealing collagen. The collagen bonding theory is also supported by our recent success in establishing argon laser welds between several collagen vascular prostheses and arteries, and by a recent report by Schober et al.[23] that revealed a homogeniz-

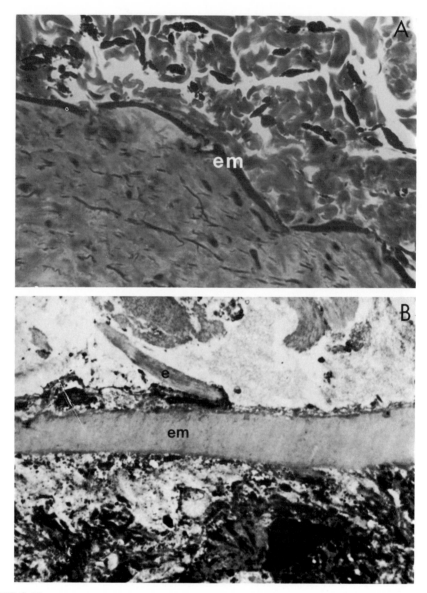

FIG 8–7.
A, histologic examination showing collagen and elastin in the media of the vein fused to internal elastic membrane *(em)* of the artery (toluidine blue, × 100). **B,** electron micrograph showing elastin *(e)* of the vein fused to denatured endothelial cells and internal elastic membrane *(em)* of artery (× 5,000). (From White RA, Kopchok G, Peng S: Laser vascular welding—How does it work? *Ann Vasc Surg,* in press. Reproduced by permission.)

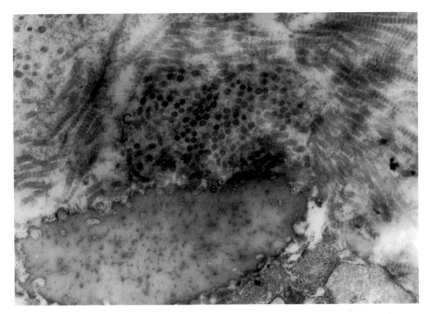

FIG 8–8.
Electron micrograph demonstrating collagen-collagen *(C)* and collagen-elastin *(e)* bonding in fusion between media of vein and adventitia of artery ($\times$ 8,000). (From White RA, Kopchok G, Peng S: Laser vascular welding—How does it work? *Ann Vasc Surg,* in press. Reproduced by permission.)

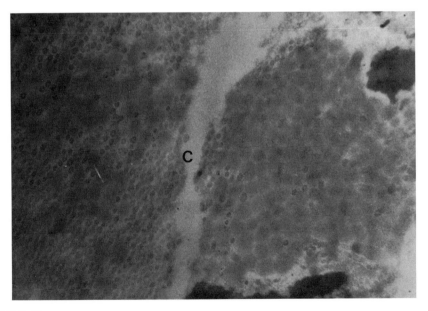

FIG 8–9.
Electron micrograph demonstrating that collagen-collagen *(C)* bonding was apparent in areas where collagen ultrastructure was swollen and blurred ($\times$ 21,000).

ing change in collagen with interdigitation of altered individual fibers that appeared to be the structural basis of the welding effect in microvessels fused with the Nd:YAG (1, 319 nm) laser.

CURRENT STATUS OF LASER VASCULAR WELDING

At present, it is known that approximation of tissue in a bloodless interface and low power (approximately 0.5 to 1 W) are required for vascular welding of medium-sized arteries by laser. Possible advantages of laser fusion over suture techniques may include healing without foreign body reaction related to sutures, preservation of mechanical properties at anastomoses, decreased intimal hyperplasia, and unrestricted enlargement of growing vessels. Possible areas for clinical use of laser fusion of vascular tissues are (1) for repairing venotomies and arteriotomies; (2) for sealing intimal flaps in endarterectomies; (3) for forming anastomoses for arteriovenous fistulas and vein-artery bypass grafts; and (4) for forming pediatric vascular anastomoses. Additional work is needed to determine the mechanism, optimal laser values, and wavelengths required for vascular tissue fusion by laser; in particular, work is needed to identify the characteristics needed to seal large-diameter arteries uniformly and to fashion welds that withstand high systemic arterial pressures. The response of both normal and diseased human vessels is also unknown, although our recent preliminary human studies using the argon laser to form Cimino arteriovenous fistulas in dialysis patients have been successful using the methodology described in this chapter.

REFERENCES

1. Dew DK, Serbent R, Hart WS, et al: Laser assisted microsurgical vessel anastomosis techniques—The use of argon and CO_2 lasers, abstracted. *Lasers Surg Med* 1983; 3:135.
2. Serure A, Withers EH, Thomsen S, et al: Comparison of carbon dioxide laser assisted microvascular anastomosis and conventional microvascular sutured anastomosis. *Surg Forum* 1984; 34:634–636.
3. Jain KK: Sutureless microvascular extra-intracranial anastomoses with Nd:YAG laser, abstracted. *Lasers Surg Med* 1984; 3:311–312.
4. Frazier OH, Painvin GA, Morris JM, et al: Laser assisted microvascular anastomoses—Angiographic and anatomopathologic studies on growing microvascular anastomoses—Preliminary report. *Surgery* 1985; 97:585–590.
5. McCarthy WJ, Hartz RS, Yao JST, et al: Vascular anastomoses with laser energy. *J Vasc Surg* 1986; 3:32–41.
6. White JV, Dalsing MC, Yao JST, et al: Tissue fusion effects of the CO_2 laser. *Surg Forum* 1985; 36:455–457.
7. Epstein M, Cooley BC: Electron microscopic study of laser dosimetry for microvascular tissue welding, abstracted. *Lasers Surg Med* 1986; 6:202.

8. White RA, Abergel RP, Klein SR, et al: Laser welding of venotomies. *Arch Surg* 1986; 121:905–907.
9. White RA, Abergel RP, Lyons R, et al: Laser welding—An alternative method of venous repair. *J Surg Res* 1986; 21:260–263.
10. White RA, Kopchok G, Donayre C, et al: Large vessel sealing with the argon laser. *Lasers Surg Med,* in press.
11. White RA, Abergel RP, Lyons R, et al: Biological effects of laser welding on vascular healing. *Lasers Surg Med* 1986; 6:137–141.
12. Ashworth EM, Dalsing M, Olson J, et al: Laser assisted vascular anastomoses of larger arteries. *Lasers Surg Med,* in press.
13. White RA, Kopchok G, Abergel RP, et al: Comparison of laser-welded and sutured arteriotomies. *Arch Surg* 1986; 121:1133–1135.
14. White RA: Technical frontiers for the vascular surgeon: Laser anastomotic welding and angioscopy assisted intraluminal instrumentation. *J Vasc Surg* 1987; 5:673–680.
15. Kopchok G, Grundfest WS, White RA, et al: Argon laser vascular welding—The thermal component. *Proc Soc Photo-Opt Instr Eng* 1986; 712:260–263.
16. Eugene J, McColgan SJ, Hammer-Wilson M, et al: Laser endarterectomy. *Lasers Surg Med* 1985; 5:265–274.
17. Eugene J, McColgan SJ, Pollock ME, et al: Experimental atherosclerosis treated by conventional and laser endarterectomy. *J Surg Res* 1985; 39:31–38.
18. Badeau AF, Lee CE, Morris JR, et al: Temperature response during microvascular anastomosis using milliwatt CO_2 laser, abstracted. *Lasers Surg Med* 1986; 6:179.
19. Quigley MR, Bailes JE, Kwaan HC, et al: Microvascular laser-assisted anastomosis—Results at one year, abstracted. *Lasers Surg Med* 1986; 2:179.
20. Quigley MR, Bailes JE, Kwaan HC, et al: Comparison of myointimal hyperplasia in laser-assisted and suture anastomosed arteries. *J Vasc Surg* 1986; 4:217–219.
21. Kopchok G, White RA, Grundfest WS, et al: Thermal studies of in-vivo vascular tissue fusion by argon laser. *Arch Surg.*
22. White RA, Kopchok G, Peng S, et al: Laser vascular welding—How does it work? *Ann Vasc Surg,* in press.
23. Schober R, Ulrich F, Sander T, et al: Laser induced alteration of collagen substructure allows microsurgical tissue welding. *Science* 1986; 232:1421–1422.

9

Future Perspectives for Angioplasty: Balloons, Lasers, and Mechanical Devices

James S. Forrester, M.D.

Warren S. Grundfest, M.D.

Frank I. Litvack, M.D.

Robert Milliken, the Nobel laureate who first measured the charge of an electron, knew a lot about the atom. In 1923 he said, "There is no likelihood man can ever top the power of the atom." Thus, a caveat: predicting is a hazardous, if necessary, business. In this final chapter, we describe the rapidly changing status of balloon angioplasty, analyze the impact of laser devices, and, finally, discuss the newest entries, an array of mechanical devices.

CURRENT STATUS OF ANGIOPLASTY

In September 1977, Andreas Gruntzig performed his first human coronary balloon angioplasty in Zurich. In less than 5 years, it became apparent that balloon angioplasty would revolutionize the management of atherosclerotic disease. In 1987, approximately 100,000 peripheral vascular dilation procedures and 115,000 coronary dilations will be performed. The National Institutes of Health expects the figures for elective coronary angioplasty to double by the year 1991. This projection does not account for patients with acute myocardial infarction who undergo combined thrombolytic therapy and balloon angioplasty.[1] Since there are approximately 650,000 patients with acute myocardial infarctions yearly in the United States, of whom perhaps 100,000 to 200,000 are potential acute angioplasty candidates, the number of coronary angioplasty procedures performed a decade from now will probably exceed 400,000 patients per year. These projections create an enormous clinical and economic impetus for the development of new and better angioplasty technology. We will not, therefore, make Robert Milliken's mistake.

STATUS OF BALLOON CATHETERS

There is still room for better technology in balloon angioplasty. Among the most interesting recent developments is the so-called balloon on a wire (the Hartzler catheter), which improves our ability to dilate distal vessels. The "monorail system," developed in Germany by Schneider Medintag Co, is a fundamental design change toward reducing the diameter of the functioning system. Clever new innovations in wire design suggest there will be a major increase in system steerability.

Nevertheless, we believe balloon technology will still have significant limitations. First, leaving room for alternate technologies, balloon systems are excellent for localized disease, in which the force of ablating an atheroma is appropriately delivered perpendicular to the long axis of the vessel. Conversely, it is not ideal for diffuse, "long-segment" disease. Second, balloons do not as yet deal effectively with total obstructions. Finally, balloon angioplasty has roughly a 30% restenosis rate. Restenosis is probably due to intimal trauma in the presence of an inadequate residual lumen. Platelet adhesion in the presence of slow flow stimulates smooth-muscle cell migration and proliferation. New devices that supplement (or less likely, replace) balloon angioplasty will, therefore, be superior in at least one of those three respects.[2]

PRESENT STATUS OF LASER ANGIOPLASTY

There are several different approaches to laser angioplasty. No one technique has emerged as clearly superior. The two best candidates, however, are the so-called hot-tip technique and the pulsed laser method.

The hot-tip is a bullet-shaped metal cap placed at the end of a fiberoptic waveguide that is rapidly heated by laser energy. Atheroma are burned away, in a manner analogous to electrocautery. The technique, admittedly crude, has already been successfully employed in man. By the end of 1986, there were reports of studies in 219 patients with peripheral vascular disease who had undergone hot-tip laser angioplasty.[3–5] The procedure is followed by balloon angioplasty. Since the procedure is still in the experimental phase, many of the patients could have had balloon angioplasty alone. Nevertheless, 51 (23%) of 219 of the lesions were classified as impossible to cross with balloons, and another 45% were considered "difficult." Of the difficult lesions, 88% were passed and followed by subsequent balloon angioplasty. Of the long-segment or total occlusions, approximately 74% were recanalized. One-year clinical follow-up is available in 74 patients. The patency rate is estimated to be 65% by clinical criteria; no follow-up angiograms have yet been reported. Based on this preliminary experience, we would predict that the hot-tip method would be an important supplement to balloon angioplasty in about 20% of cases and would be best for total obstructions and long-segment disease in large vessels.

The experience in clinical coronary disease comes from anecdotal reports (such as letters to the editor[6] and an addendum[7]). Thermal laser angioplasty has been attempted in 14 human coronary vessels. It was successfully completed in six. In four patients the probe could not be passed across the lesion. There was one perforation; three additional patients suffered either myocardial infarction or vessel occlusion within hours of the procedure.

These earliest data establish the feasibility of percutaneous hot-tip laser angioplasty, but not, as yet, its long-term efficacy. As of March 1, 1987, this technology has FDA approval for peripheral artery applications. Strategies for improving this technology include methods for monitoring the tip temperature, better tips, and guidance systems. If the hot-tip method is successful, it is also likely that a less expensive energy source than lasers will be developed.

PULSED LASERS

Pulsed lasers have an advantage that may become the solution to thrombus formation following hot-tip ablation; they vaporize tissue yet cause minimal burn injury. At Cedars-Sinai Medical Center Los Angeles, our preference among pulsed lasers is the ultraviolet laser, because we believe it combines the greatest precision with the ability to cut through calcified material. Among the ultraviolet laser group, we prefer the 308-nm excimer laser, because it is readily transmitted through fiberoptics. At present, we are awaiting FDA approval to begin intraoperative trials of peripheral vascular excimer laser angioplasty.

The laser angioplasty field is burgeoning with innovations. At the Massachusetts Institute of Technology, Cambridge, Michael Feld, Ph.D. and his colleagues are using differences in the patterns of laser-induced fluorescence to distinguish atheromatous from normal vascular tissue.[8] This laser operates in the millisecond range. Fully developed, this "smart laser" would first analyze its target biochemically before deciding to fire. By using multiple fibers, it would be possible to create "tiny nibbles" in the atheroma with each pulse. No clinical results have yet been obtained with this system. Other groups are investigating sapphire-capped fibers[9] as an alternative to the metal hot-tip. Although no particular advantage of this technology has been demonstrated, it is an indication of the array of potential solutions that are being actively considered.

ALTERNATIVE MECHANICAL TECHNOLOGIES

The recognition that blood flow can be safely restored by intravascular intervention has led other groups to investigate mechanical devices. At present, the two most interesting devices are the Kensey rotating cam and the Simpson "atherectomy" catheter. The Kensey catheter contains within it a cam that rotates at 100,000 rpm, creating a vortex of accelerated fluid around it. Micropellets of high-velocity fluid are driven laterally against the vessel wall, while the cam drills forward along the long axis. The device has been used to date in approximately 50 human peripheral vessels. Patency was achieved in about 85%; the long-term patency rate is not yet established.[10] An alternative drill system developed by Auth and Richie has a tip studded with 30-μm diamonds, which are cooled by a saline flush. Intuitively, we would expect drills to be plagued by downstream embolization. Remarkably, this has not been a recognizable clinical problem in peripheral vessels.

If a drill is not successful, perhaps a tiny catheter-mounted blade, designed to excise the atheroma, may be a solution. The Simpson atherectomy catheter is the prototype device for this approach. The device produces dramatic angiographic improvement in short-segment peripheral vascular disease. To date, the atherectomy catheter has been used in 89 peripheral vessels and was successful in opening the artery in 87[11]; however, adequate long-term follow-up is not yet available. The major problem with use of mechanical devices for coronary and small-vessel applications may become the inability to miniaturize them below a certain level.

If it is not possible to predict which (if any) of this spectacular array of new technologies will be used and which will be discarded, we can confidently predict that, in the long view of history, this will be the decade in which intravascular intervention comes of age. And we can avoid the error of Charles Duell, director of the U.S. Patent Office in 1899, who recommended closing the office, with the observation that "everything that can be invented has been invented."

REFERENCES

1. Topol EJ, Califf RM, George BS: A multicenter randomized trial of intravenous recombinant tissue plasminogen activator and emergency coronary angioplasty for acute myocardial infarction: Preliminary report from the Tami study, abstracted. *Circulation* 1986; 74(suppl 2):23.
2. Forrester JS, Litvack F, Grundfest W, et al: A perspective of coronary disease seen through the arteries of living man *Circulation* 1987; 75:505–513.
3. Sanborn TA, Cumberland DC, Greenfield AJ, et al: Six month follow-up on laserprobe assisted balloon angioplasty, abstracted. *Circulation* 1986; 74(suppl 2):457
4. Sanborn TA, Greenfield AJ, Guben JK, et al: Human percutaneous and intraopera-

tive laser thermal angioplasty—Initial clinical results as an adjunct to balloon angioplasty. *J Vasc Surg* 1987; 5:183–190.

5. Cumberland DC, Sanborn TA, Taylor DI, et al: Percutaneous laser thermal angioplasty—Initial clinical results with a laserprobe in total peripheral artery occlusions. *Lancet* 1986; 1:1457–1459.

6. Cumberland DC, Starkey IR, Oakley GDG: Percutaneous laser-assisted coronary angioplasty. *Lancet* 1986; 1:214.

7. Sanborn TA, Faxon DP, Kellett MA, et al: Percutaneous coronary laser thermal angioplasty. *J Am Coll Cardiol* 1986; 8:1437–1440.

8. Cothren RM, Hayes GB, Cramer JR, et al: A multifiber catheter with an optical shield for laser angiosurgery. *Lasers Life Sci* 1987; 1:1–12.

9. Fourrier JL, Marache P, Brunetaud J, et al: Laser recanalization of peripheral arteries by contact sapphire in man, abstracted. *Circulation* 1986; 74(suppl 2):204.

10. Kensey K: Personal communication, March 1987.

11. Simpson JB, Zimmerman JJ, Matthews R, et al: Transluminal atherectomy: Initial clinical results in 27 patients, abstracted. *Circulation* 1986; 74(suppl 2):203.

Index